AUTOMATED EXTERNAL DEFIBRILLATION

James W. Drake

University of Mississippi Medical Center

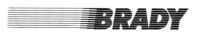

Brady/Prentice Hall
Upper Saddle River, NJ 07458

Library of Congress Cataloging-in-Publication Data

Drake, James W.
    Automated external defibrillation / James Drake.
        p.   cm.
    ISBN 0-13-084383-0 (pkb. : alk. paper)
    1. Electric countershock. 2. Defibrillators. 3. Cardiac arrest.
    I. Title.
    RC684.E4D73   1999
    616.1′23025—dc21   99-38345
                                                        CIP

Publisher: *Julie Alexander*
Acquisitions Editor: *Judy Streger*
Director of Production and Manufacturing: *Bruce Johnson*
Managing Production Editor: *Patrick Walsh*
Senior Production Manager: *Ilene Sanford*
Production Liaison: *Danielle Newhouse*
Production Editor: *Susan Geraghty*
Creative Director: *Marianne Frasco*
Interior Designer: *Publishers' Design and Production Services, Inc.*
Cover Designer: *Jayne Conte*
Cover Photographer: *Tony Stone Images/ Jon Riley*
Marketing Manager: *Tiffany Price*
Marketing Coordinator: *Cindy Frederick*
Composition: *Publishers' Design and Production Services, Inc.*
Printing and Binding: *R. R. Donnelley & Sons*

© 2000 by Prentice-Hall, Inc.
Upper Saddle River, New Jersey 07458

Printed in the United States of America

10 9 8 7 6 5 4 3 2 1

ISBN 0-13-084383-0

Prentice-Hall International (UK) Limited, *London*
Prentice-Hall of Australia Pty. Limited, *Sydney*
Prentice-Hall Canada Inc., *Toronto*
Prentice-Hall Hispanoamericana, S.A., *Mexico*
Prentice-Hall of India Private Limited:, *New Delhi*
Prentice-Hall of Japan, Inc., *Tokyo*
Prentice-Hall Singapore Pty. Ltd.
Editoria Prentice-Hall do Brasil, Ltda., *Rio de Janeiro*

Notice: The author and the publisher of this book have taken care to make certain that the equipment and schedules of treatment are correct and compatible with the standards generally accepted at the time of publication. Nevertheless, as new information becomes available, changes in treatment and in the use of equipment and procedures become necessary. The reader is advised to consult carefully the instruction and information material included in each piece of equipment or device before administration. Students are warned that the use of any techniques must be authorized by their medical advisor, where appropriate, in accordance with local laws and regulations. The publisher disclaims any liability, loss, injury, or damage incurred as a consequence, directly or indirectly, of the use and application of any of the contents of this book.

Contents

Preface

Every year, more than 250,000 people in the United States suffer sudden cardiac arrest (American Heart Association, 1998). Sudden cardiac arrest occurs when the heart unexpectedly loses its ability to pump blood through the body. Without blood circulating throughout the body, a person will quickly die. Sudden cardiac arrest can occur anywhere—at home, on an airplane, in a shopping mall, while traveling on a desolate stretch of highway, or on a crowded street corner.

For many, sudden cardiac arrest quickly becomes cardiac death. Nevertheless, there are those who survive sudden cardiac arrest. Why do some die but others survive? The secret is simple: early defibrillation.

Early defibrillation can restore a heartbeat and allow the heart to again pump oxygen-rich blood throughout the body. However, if defibrillation is to be successful, it must occur within the first few minutes of cardiac arrest.

In the past, few people were certified to provide early defibrillation. Extensive training was needed to learn the different electrical rhythms of the heart and which patients would benefit from a defibrillating shock. The lack of certified providers increased the time it took to get a defibrillator to a patient's side. Usually, by the time a defibrillator did arrive, too much time had passed, and defibrillation was no longer an option. As a result, there was little hope for the person in cardiac arrest.

Fortunately, this picture is changing. Technological advances have produced a new generation of automated external defibrillators (AEDs). AEDs are machines that automatically analyze a cardiac arrest patient's heart and deliver a defibrillating shock when needed. The computerized device eliminates the need for extensive training. Indeed, the AED has made defibrillation so simple that even people with no medical background can easily learn to administer it and save a cardiac arrest patient's life. Because of AEDs, early defibrillation can be brought to the cardiac arrest patient's side faster than ever before.

The American Heart Association has initiated a program called *Public Access Defibrillation*. The goal of this program is to extend the AED's early defibrillation capability to the greatest number of people possible. The American Heart Association has identified several groups of people who are most likely to first reach a cardiac arrest patient's side and provide early defibrillation with the AED. These groups include firefighters, lifeguards, police officers, security guards, flight attendants, and family members of high-risk cardiac patients. Because learning to use the AED is so simple, even laypeople with no medical background may be able to provide early defibrillation (American Heart Association, 1997).

The goal of this book is to support the idea of public access to defibrillation and to increase the survivability of sudden cardiac arrest. To accomplish this goal, the book discusses how to provide emergency cardiac treatment using an AED. Additionally, it is hoped that once the AED's simplicity and effectiveness become apparent, interest in developing community-wide early defibrillation programs will follow.

ACKNOWLEDGMENTS

The author would like to thank the following individuals for their time and effort in reviewing the material and making invaluable suggestions and contributions.

Chad E. Jarvis, CCEMT-P
Emergency Medical Services Program
   Coordinator
Randolph Community College
Asheboro, North Carolina

Chuck Carter, RN, CEN, NREMT-P
Basic Life Support Coordinator
Mississippi State Department of
   Health
Division of Emergency Medical
   Services
Jackson, Mississippi

Don Whiteley, Jr.
Manager for Training and
   Certification
South Carolina Office of Emergency
   Medical Services
Columbia, South Carolina

Helen Yurong, MSN, EMT-P
Nurse Educator and EMT Instructor
Naval Medical Clinic
Pearl Harbor, Hawaii

Sue Archer, RNC
Health Occupations Instructor
Mingo Job Corps CCC
Puxico, Missouri

Robert D. Cook, EMT-P, I/C
St. Johns Regional Health Center
Springfield, Missouri

Lee Burns
New York State Department of
   Health
Bureau of EMS
Saratoga Emergency Medical Services
Saratoga Springs, New York

Jo Anne Schultz, BA, NREMT-P
Salisbury Emergency Medical Services
Maryland Fire and Rescue Institute
Salisbury, Maryland

**Gail A. Stewart, EMS Programs
  Coordinator**
Santa Fe Community College
Gainesville, Florida

Mark J. Reis, NREMT-P
Education Coordinator
Acadian Ambulance and Air Medical
  Services
Lafayette, Louisiana

**Steven B. Engish, RN, CCRN,
  EMT-B**
Careflight
St. Joseph's Hospital
Lexington, Kentucky

Richard Ellis, NREMT-P, AAS
Texas

Lt. Rudy Garrett
Training Coordinator
Somerset-Pulaski County EMS
Somerset, Kentucky

REFERENCES

American Heart Association. (1997). *Basic life support for healthcare providers.*
  Dallas: Author.
American Heart Association. (1998). *Heartsaver AED for the lay rescuer and first
  responder.* Dallas: Author.

Introduction

John Maynerd, a sixty-three-year-old new retiree, is running errands this Friday morning. He enjoys the crisp autumn air as he stops at the bank to deposit his first pension check. John is planning to give a surprise birthday party in one week for his wife of forty-one years. All of their children and grandchildren will be there. For the first time in three years, everyone will be together under one roof. Life could not be better. Or could it?

When John awoke this morning, he did not feel quite himself. While walking to the bathroom, he noticed he was somewhat short of breath. Also, he was sweating, even though he was not hot. Eventually the shortness of breath and sweating passed, and he again felt normal. Strangely, though, the shortness of breath and sweating have now returned, in the bank. In addition, John notices a feeling of pressure in his chest.

Two weeks ago, John visited his doctor for a preretirement physical. The doctor pointed out that John's blood pressure was high and he needed to take his daily medications as prescribed. Unfortunately, John discounted his doctor's advice, as he felt that his blood pressure, even though high, was not causing him any problems. He assured himself that he was fine.

"Oh, well," John thought, "it is probably just fatigue from planning this surprise party." After all, being newly retired, he was enjoying life. Nothing bad could happen. Still, he was somewhat worried, and he resolved to begin taking his blood pressure medication as prescribed in the morning.

"Good morning, Mister Maynerd!" greets Elizabeth, the bank teller.

Everyone knows John; his is a familiar face around town, and he has been a loyal bank customer for twenty-two years. He looks at Elizabeth and attempts to reply. He can't. His thoughts are not making sense. . . . He can't breath. . . . He can't think. He finds himself sweating heavily and having a harder time breathing.

"Mister Maynerd, are you okay?" inquires Elizabeth as she observes the color leave his face.

The teller goes in and out of focus. John mumbles a few incomprehensible words and becomes very dizzy. Suddenly, he gets very tired and his world goes black. . . .

Bank patrons hear John expel a loud grunt, and then he collapses to the floor.

"*Someone call an ambulance!*" shouts Elizabeth as she quickly makes her way to John's side.

The bank manager promptly picks up the telephone and dials 911. After reporting the situation, the 911 dispatcher informs the manager that an ambulance is being dispatched and paramedics will be there in fifteen minutes. Because of the long response time, the dispatcher is also notifying the police department. The police officers in this community have been specially trained as first responders and can administer emergency medical care until the paramedics arrive. The dispatcher then instructs the manager to have someone assess John for responsiveness, breathing, and a pulse.

Elizabeth assesses John and finds him unresponsive, breathless, and without a pulse. Based on this information, the dispatcher informs the bank manager that John's heart has stopped beating—that he is in cardiac arrest. The dispatcher asks if anyone at the bank can perform CPR. The manager quickly repeats this question to all of those present.

"I took a CPR class about a year ago. I think I can remember," an older woman states.

Nervously, she approaches John and begins to perform CPR. Even though she is rusty, the correct sequence for delivering rescue breaths and chest compressions quickly comes back to her.

The bank falls silent. For all involved, time appears to stand still. Although the paramedics are still about twelve minutes away, the distant wail of an approaching police car is heard.

Will CPR keep John alive until the police and paramedics arrive? Will the police have an automated external defibrillator? If an automated external defibrillator is available, will defibrillation occur in time? Will his wife's surprise party be supplanted by a funeral?

1

The Heart
and Cardiac Arrest

LEARNING OBJECTIVES

At the end of this chapter, you will be able to

- Describe the location of the heart
- Describe the function of the heart
- Define cardiac arrest
- Identify the three signs of cardiac arrest

KEY TERMS

Heart—A fist-sized muscular organ that pumps blood throughout the body.

Cells—Tiny living building blocks that make up all human beings.

Oxygen—Odorless, tasteless, colorless gas necessary for life. All cells require oxygen for survival.

Cardiac arrest—A condition in which the heart ceases to pump blood.

To provide effective emergency cardiac care, you must first understand the heart and how it functions. It is also important to understand the condition of cardiac arrest, since this is what the AED is designed to correct. Accordingly, this chapter discusses the heart's location and function and the condition and effects of cardiac arrest.

LOCATION OF THE HEART

The **heart** is a fist-sized, muscular organ located in the chest. More specifically, the heart lies behind and to the left of the breastbone, or **sternum** (see Figure 1–1). Knowledge of the heart's location is important when applying an AED to a person in cardiac arrest. (Physical application of the AED is discussed in Chapter Four.)

FUNCTION OF THE HEART

The heart pumps blood to and from the **cells** of the body. The human body is made up of trillions of tiny living cells. These cells form the organs—the brain, heart, lungs, kidneys, and so on—that perform the vital functions that give us life. For cells and organs to survive, they must receive a continuous supply of **oxygen**, transported by the blood.

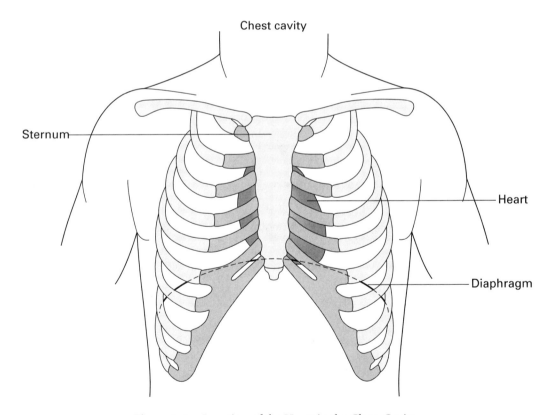

Figure 1–1   Location of the Heart in the Chest Cavity

The heart is divided into two sides: the left and the right. As we breathe, oxygen enters the lungs. Once in the lungs, the oxygen is transferred onto red blood cells, creating oxygen-rich blood. With every beat of the heart, this oxygen-rich blood is pumped by the left side of the heart into large blood vessels called **arteries.** From the arteries, the oxygen-rich blood is forced into **capillaries.** Capillaries are tiny blood vessels that lie next to cells.

Where the capillaries and cells meet, oxygen leaves the bloodstream and enters the cells for their internal use. The blood, now depleted of oxygen, continues on, traveling through the body's **veins** until it reaches the right side of the heart. The right side of the heart then pumps the oxygen-poor blood back into the lungs for reoxygenation. At this point, the entire cycle starts over again with the left side of the heart (see Figure 1–2).

This cycle represents the most basic process of life. Without a beating heart, oxygen-rich blood is not circulated to the cells. Without oxygen, cells and organs will quickly die. Without living organs, a person cannot survive.

CARDIAC COMPROMISE

When a problem arises with the heart and its ability to pump blood, **cardiac** (heart) **compromise** occurs. A **heart attack,** or **acute myocardial infarction** (*acute* means "sudden"; *myocardial* refers to heart muscle; *infarction* means "death"), is the most common form of cardiac compromise. A heart attack occurs when a significant number of the cells that make up the heart suddenly die. If enough of these cells die, the heart can lose its ability to pump blood throughout the body to the waiting cells.

A person suffering a heart attack typically complains of dull or crushing chest pain. The chest pain may be accompanied by other symptoms, such as nausea, shortness of breath, arm pain, weakness, and sweating.

The effects of a heart attack can be mild to severe. On the one hand, a person suffering a mild heart attack may not experience any discomfort and may never even realize he or she has sustained one! On the other hand, some heart attacks are so severe that cardiac arrest quickly follows.

CARDIAC ARREST

Cardiac arrest (*cardiac* refers to the heart; *arrest* means "stop") occurs when the heart suddenly stops pumping blood. Typically, cardiac arrest occurs after the onset of warning signs like chest pain or shortness of breath. However, cardiac arrest may occur without any warning signs and thus become the first and only

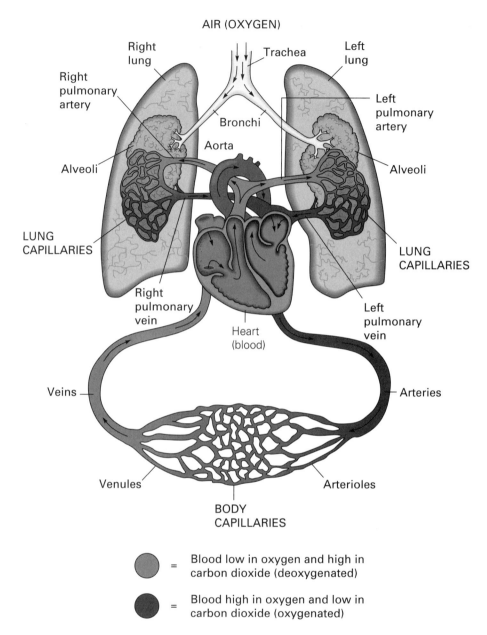

Figure 1–2 Blood Circulation Through the Cardiovascular System (*Source:* Hafen, Karren, & Mistovich, 1996, p. 295)

indication of a heart problem. Because the heart in cardiac arrest loses its ability to pump blood, oxygen is not circulated to the awaiting cells.

The brain and the heart itself are both especially sensitive to losing oxygen-rich blood. After four minutes of being deprived of oxygen, brain cells are damaged. If brain cells go ten minutes without oxygen-rich blood, they die and brain death occurs. When the brain dies, it loses the ability to control the many internal functions that give us life.

The cells of the heart are no different. After ten minutes of not receiving oxygen-rich blood, the heart becomes extremely difficult to revive. For this reason, time is of the essence when providing emergency care to a person in cardiac arrest.

Aside from heart attacks, cardiac arrest can be caused by massive blood loss, electrocution, poisoning, choking, and drowning. Regardless of the cause, a heart in cardiac arrest loses its ability to pump oxygen-rich blood to the cells of the body. If circulation is not restored, the person in cardiac arrest will die.

A person in cardiac arrest displays three signs: unresponsiveness, breathlessness, and a lack of pulse. As the supply of oxygen-rich blood to the brain is lost, so is the brain's ability to maintain a state of consciousness or responsiveness. Therefore, the person in cardiac arrest will be unresponsive.

The brain controls breathing by signaling the lungs to inflate and deflate. A dying brain cannot send these signals, and thus breathing will not occur. Therefore, the person in cardiac arrest will be breathless.

Finally, since his or her heart cannot pump blood, a patient in cardiac arrest will not have a pulse. (Pulses and assessing for a pulse are presented in Chapter Five.)

SUMMARY

Learning to provide emergency care for a person in cardiac arrest starts with acquiring a basic knowledge of the heart and its function. To stay alive, we must have a beating heart that circulates oxygen-rich blood to the cells of our body.

In a person in cardiac arrest, the heart stops pumping blood and oxygen is not delivered to the awaiting cells. Without oxygen, these cells become damaged and will die if circulation is not restored. This is especially true for the cells of the heart and brain.

Quick delivery of emergency care can reverse cardiac arrest by restoring the heart's ability to circulate oxygen-rich blood to the body's cells. If circulation is restored before the brain, heart, and other organs die, the person in cardiac arrest stands a good chance of surviving. This is the goal in providing emergency care to a person in cardiac arrest.

FOOD FOR THOUGHT

To test your understanding, read and discuss the following questions.

1. *Where is the heart located? What is its basic function?*

   The heart is located in the chest, behind and just to the left of the breastbone, or sternum. Look at yourself and envision where your heart lies. The basic function of the heart is to pump oxygen-rich blood to the cells of the body and then return oxygen-poor blood back to the lungs for reoxygenation. Once reoxygenated, the blood is recirculated to the cells of the body.

2. *Why is a beating heart necessary for life?*

   The human body is made up of trillions of tiny cells, which form organs that perform vital functions to give us life. All cells require oxygen to live. A beating heart pumps oxygen-rich blood to the cells. If the heart does not pump blood, oxygen is not circulated to the cells. If deprived of oxygen, the cells of the body will die. When cells die, so do the organs that they form. Without living organs, a person cannot survive.

3. *What happens to the heart and its ability to pump blood when a person suffers cardiac arrest? Why is this dangerous to the human body?*

   Cardiac arrest occurs when the heart loses its ability to pump blood. Since blood is not circulated throughout the body, the cells do not receive oxygen. Remember that cells cannot survive without oxygen and will eventually die if deprived of it. When cells die, so do the organs that they make up. The cells of the brain and heart quickly die in the absence of oxygen-rich blood. After ten minutes of being denied oxygen-rich blood, brain death occurs, and the heart becomes very difficult to resuscitate. When a person's brain, heart, and other organs die, a person cannot survive.

4. *A person in cardiac arrest presents with three distinct signs. Describe these three signs and explain why they occur in people in cardiac arrest.*

   A person in cardiac arrest is unresponsive, breathless, and without a pulse. Without oxygen-rich blood, the brain quickly becomes dysfunctional and loses its ability to maintain a state of consciousness. Therefore, the person in cardiac arrest will be unresponsive. Also, the dysfunctional brain cannot send messages to the lungs to inflate and deflate. Consequently, the person in cardiac arrest will be breathless. Finally, as the heart has ceased pumping blood, the person in cardiac arrest will not have a pulse.

REFERENCES

Hafen, B. Q., Karren, K. J., & Mistovich, J. J. (1996). *Prehospital emergency care* (5th ed.). Upper Saddle River, NJ: Prentice Hall.

Weigel, A., Atkins, J. M., & Taylor, J. (1988). *Automated defibrillation*. Englewood, CO: Morton Publishing.

C H A P T E R

2

Emergency Care
and Cardiac Arrest

LEARNING OBJECTIVES

At the end of this chapter, you will be able to

- Describe the four critical actions of emergency cardiac care
- Describe the interdependency that exists between the four critical actions of emergency cardiac care
- Describe the problem of providing early defibrillation
- Describe how defibrillation and the AED fit into the overall scheme of emergency cardiac care

KEY TERMS

Cardiopulmonary resuscitation (CPR)—Delivery of rescue breathing and chest compressions to a person in cardiac arrest.

Defibrillation—Controlled delivery of electrical shocks to a heart in cardiac arrest. Frequently, early defibrillation serves to restart the heart, enabling it to pump blood.

Automated external defibrillator (AED)—A device capable of automatically delivering defibrillation. An AED requires little training to operate.

Chain of Survival—A sequence, developed by the American Heart Association, consisting of the four critical actions (links in the chain) that must be taken to give a cardiac arrest patient the best chance for survival.

Cardiac arrest occurs when the heart stops pumping blood. If a person is to survive cardiac arrest, four critical actions must quickly be performed. These four actions make up emergency care for the cardiac arrest patient and are described in this chapter. The chapter also introduces the AED and its role in emergency cardiac care.

The Chain of Survival

The American Heart Association has identified four critical actions that, when performed quickly, increase a person's chance of surviving cardiac arrest (American Heart Association, 1997). Collectively, these four critical actions form the **Chain of Survival.**

For the person in cardiac arrest, the Chain of Survival represents their greatest hope for recovery. The four actions, or "links," in the chain are

1. *Early access.* This term is used to describe the recognition of a cardiac emergency and quick notification of the emergency medical services (EMS) system. Once notified, specially trained personnel and equipment are summoned to the cardiac patient's location. Dialing 911 or other appropriate emergency telephone number activates most EMS systems. *The earlier access occurs, the sooner help will arrive, and the better the patient's chance for survival!* If access is delayed or does not occur at all, a cardiac arrest patient's opportunity for survival significantly decreases.

2. *Early CPR.* CPR temporarily substitutes rescue breaths and chest compressions for the lost functions of breathing and a beating heart. Artificially inflating the patient's lungs and compressing his or her chest allows blood to be oxygenated and circulated to the cells of the brain, heart, and other organs until corrective measures like defibrillation and advanced care can arrive. Without early CPR, the cells of the brain, heart, and other organs may die, making resuscitation very difficult.

3. *Early defibrillation.* **Defibrillation** is the controlled delivery of electrical shocks to a heart in cardiac arrest. As explained in Chapter Three, defibrillating shock may restart the heart, enabling it once again to pump oxygen-rich blood to the cells of the body. The AED is a device that automatically performs defibrillation. *For defibrillation to be effective, it must be delivered early on!* Remember, after four minutes of cardiac arrest, the oxygen-deprived cells of the brain and heart become damaged. After ten minutes, a significant portion of the heart and brain die, making resuscitation very difficult, even with defibrillation.

CPR can preserve the heart and brain by artificially perfusing them with oxygen-rich blood. As such, CPR delays cells from dying and increases the time period in which successful defibrillation can occur.

4. *Early advanced care.* **Advanced care** consists of procedures like controlling the patient's airway, administering IV fluids or drugs, and defibrillation if it has not yet been performed. Both those who have responded to defibrillation and those who have not require early advanced care. Doctors, nurses, and paramedics are capable of providing advanced care.

Like any chain, the Chain of Survival's strength depends on all of its links working together. A weak or missing link weakens the chain and limits the patient's opportunity for survival. If a patient does not receive early CPR or early defibrillation, early advanced care can do very little to save him or her. Similarly, early access and early CPR are futile if early defibrillation and early advanced care are not available. To make cardiac arrest survivable, all four links must be strong and performed as quickly as possible.

THE AED'S PLACE IN THE CHAIN OF SURVIVAL

In the past, early defibrillation was a weak link in the Chain of Survival. Before the invention of the AED, extensive training was required to administer defibrillation. Consequently, few people were certified to deliver this life-saving skill. Frequently, too much time passed before a person in cardiac arrest received a defibrillating shock. Despite early recognition and early CPR, defibrillation was often no longer an option by the time it could be performed. Survival rates for cardiac arrest were thus extremely poor.

The development of the AED tremendously strengthened this weak link. AEDs have simplified the training required to deliver this life-saving procedure, making defibrillation more accessible to those who require it. Combined with the remaining three links, AEDs have strengthened the Chain of Survival and increased people's chances of surviving cardiac arrest.

SUMMARY

A person's best chance for surviving cardiac arrest is when all four "links" in the Chain of Survival are strong and support one another. A weak or missing link weakens the chain and decreases a cardiac arrest patient's chance for survival.

Just as single links do not form a chain, the individual measures of emergency cardiac care, by themselves, are not effective in saving a cardiac arrest patient's life. All measures of emergency cardiac care are important in the resuscitation effort.

FOOD FOR THOUGHT

To test your understanding, read and discuss the following questions.

1. *You have been summoned to a cardiac arrest patient's side but do not have an AED available for use. To give the patient his or her best opportunity for survival, what can you do until an AED arrives?*

   CPR must be performed until an AED arrives. CPR will artificially oxygenate the blood and circulate it to the body's cells. As a result, organs like the brain and heart will be preserved until the heart can be successfully defibrillated and once again pump oxygen-rich blood to the body.

2. *Identify the four links in the Chain of Survival and discuss their importance in providing emergency care for a person in cardiac arrest. What is a person's chance for surviving cardiac arrest if any of these links are weak or missing?*

   The four links in the Chain of Survival are early access, early CPR, early defibrillation, and early advanced care. Early access gets the system moving by recognizing the cardiac emergency and summoning specialized help to the patient's side. Early CPR preserves the cells of the body by artificially circulating oxygen-rich blood. If delivered early enough, defibrillation can restart the heart. Finally, early advanced care provides procedures and drugs that can help a person whose heart has been restarted by defibrillation or a person whose heart will not respond to a defibrillating shock.

   If any of these links are missing or weak, the opportunity for surviving cardiac arrest decreases tremendously. If early access does not occur, the person will never have the chance for early CPR, early defibrillation, or early advanced care. If early access does occur but early CPR or early defibrillation are not provided, survival is extremely difficult. Remember that for a person to survive cardiac arrest, all four links must be strong and performed without delay.

3. *Why was the delivery of early defibrillation severely limited prior to the development of the AED?*

   Before the AED, becoming certified to deliver emergency defibrillation required extensive training in cardiac rhythm interpretation and operation of the defibrillator. As a result, few people were able to deliver the life-saving skill. This weakened the link of early defibrillation and decreased the survivability of cardiac arrest.

4. *Why has the AED strengthened the Chain of Survival and bettered a person's chances for surviving cardiac arrest?*

Because they are automated, AEDs have eliminated the extensive training requirements previously associated with defibrillation and have simplified the process of administering defibrillation. This has made defibrillation more accessible, both to those who deliver it and to those who require it. Therefore, the previously weak link of early defibrillation has been strengthened, and the likelihood of surviving cardiac arrest is greater than ever before.

REFERENCES

American Heart Association. (1997). *Basic life support for healthcare providers.* Dallas: Author.

Hafen, B. Q., Karren, K. J., & Mistovich, J. J. (1996). *Prehospital emergency care* (5th ed.). Upper Saddle River, NJ: Prentice Hall.

3

Defibrillation and Cardiac Arrest

LEARNING OBJECTIVES

At the end of this chapter, you will be able to

- Describe defibrillation
- Describe why defibrillation is important in treating cardiac arrest
- Describe why defibrillation must occur early on

KEY TERMS

Shockable cardiac arrest—A state of cardiac arrest that will benefit from early defibrillation.

Nonshockable cardiac arrest—A state of cardiac arrest that will not benefit from a defibrillating shock.

Ventricular fibrillation—The most common form of shockable cardiac arrest. Ventricular fibrillation often responds to early defibrillation.

Early defibrillation is a critical link in the Chain of Survival. If a person is to survive cardiac arrest, early defibrillation must occur. This chapter introduces defibrillation and its role in emergency cardiac care.

DEFIBRILLATION

Defibrillation is the controlled delivery of electrical shocks to a heart that has stopped pumping blood. The sudden surge of electricity from a defibrillator "resets" the heart and restores the heartbeat, allowing the heart to once again pump oxygen-rich blood throughout the body.

Unfortunately, not everyone in cardiac arrest will benefit from a defibrillating shock. A heart in cardiac arrest is classified as either shockable or nonshockable. A heart in a shockable state may benefit from a defibrillating shock, but a heart in a nonshockable state will not. With an AED, you do not have to decide whether the heart is shockable or nonshockable—the AED will automatically analyze the heart and inform you of whether or not it is shockable.

Shockable Cardiac Arrest

At the onset of cardiac arrest, the heart typically goes into a condition called **ventricular fibrillation,** a state in which the heart quivers weakly like a glob of gelatin (*ventricular* refers to the lower portion of the heart; *fibrillation* refers to disorganized, feeble contractions). This quivering action is not a heartbeat. The weak chaotic motion of a heart experiencing ventricular fibrillation is incapable of pumping blood; therefore, ventricular fibrillation results in cardiac arrest. When an AED detects ventricular fibrillation, it will identify the heart as shockable and advise you to prepare for immediate defibrillation.

Early defibrillation can terminate the quivering action of ventricular fibrillation and restore a heartbeat that is capable of pumping blood. If ventricular fibrillation does not receive early defibrillation, the quivering action will eventually cease, and the heart will become completely still. Often referred to as the **flat-line** or by the term **asystole,** this state of cardiac arrest is nonshockable and most often signifies a dead heart.

Nonshockable Cardiac Arrest

The heart in a nonshockable state of cardiac arrest will not benefit from a defibrillating shock. An AED will automatically identify nonshockable cardiac arrest and advise you of its presence. When nonshockable cardiac arrest is present, the AED will not let the rescuer shock the patient. Nonshockable cardiac arrest is best treated with CPR and advanced care.

The Importance of Acting Early On

Defibrillation can never occur too early! Three principles illustrate the importance of early defibrillation:

- Ventricular fibrillation is the most frequently occurring state of the heart immediately following the onset of cardiac arrest.

- A defibrillating shock is the most effective way to stop ventricular fibrillation and produce a heartbeat capable of circulating oxygen-rich blood to the cells and organs of the body.
- Ventricular fibrillation becomes less responsive to defibrillation with each passing minute. The shockable state of ventricular fibrillation degenerates into a nonshockable state in about ten minutes. Nonshockable cardiac arrest will not respond to defibrillation. In a nonshockable state the heart is no longer fibrillating (it is still), and thus it cannot be *de*fibrillated (American Heart Association, 1997).

As a rule, the chances of successfully converting ventricular fibrillation into a regular heartbeat with a defibrillating shock decrease by 10 percent with each passing minute. Subsequently, the best chance for conversion is when the patient is defibrillated during the first minute following cardiac arrest (90 percent chance for conversion). If defibrillation has not occurred after nine minutes, there is only a 10 percent chance for successful conversion. After ten minutes, nonshockable cardiac arrest is most often encountered (Mistovitch, Benner, & Margolis, 1998). Thus defibrillation is most effective when performed *early on.* Any delay in the delivery of defibrillating shock can mean the difference between life and death.

As discussed in Chapter Two, successful defibrillation also depends on the other links in the Chain of Survival. If early access is delayed or does not occur, time passes and the opportunity for successful defibrillation diminishes. Additionally, early advanced care is critical for all cardiac arrest patients—both those who have had their heartbeat restored by defibrillation and those who have entered a state of nonshockable cardiac arrest.

As discussed previously, CPR can temporarily extend the time period in which successful defibrillation may occur. By perfusing the heart cells with oxygen-rich blood, CPR can allow the heart to remain responsive to defibrillation for a longer period of time. However, CPR can rarely by itself restore a heartbeat to a heart experiencing ventricular fibrillation. Therefore, even if CPR is being administered, defibrillation must occur at the earliest possible moment.

Summary

Cardiac arrest occurs in two forms—shockable cardiac arrest and nonshockable cardiac arrest. Shockable cardiac arrest can benefit from the delivery of a defibrillating shock; nonshockable cardiac arrest cannot. Conveniently, an AED automatically analyzes a patient's heart and advises you of whether shockable or nonshockable cardiac arrest is present. If shockable cardiac arrest exists, the AED will prepare to deliver a shock. If a nonshockable form of cardiac arrest is identified, the AED will not allow you to shock the patient.

Ventricular fibrillation is a shockable form of cardiac arrest, found in the majority of patients immediately following the onset of cardiac arrest. Ventricular fibrillation is most effectively converted to a productive heartbeat through early defibrillation. Unfortunately, a heart experiencing ventricular fibrillation becomes less and less responsive to defibrillation with each passing minute. After ten minutes, the shockable state of cardiac arrest most often turns into a nonshockable state, for which defibrillation holds no benefit. Therefore, defibrillation of a person in shockable cardiac arrest can never occur too early!

FOOD FOR THOUGHT

To test your understanding, read and discuss the following questions.

1. *For defibrillation to be effective at restoring a heartbeat, it must occur as quickly as possible following the onset of cardiac arrest. Why must it occur early on?*

   At the onset of cardiac arrest, the heart most frequently enters a shockable state called ventricular fibrillation. The longer that state persists, the more difficult it becomes to successfully defibrillate the heart—to convert the fibrillation into a regular heartbeat. Eventually, the shockable state of ventricular fibrillation will degenerate into a nonshockable form of cardiac arrest for which defibrillation holds no benefit.

   Remember that the chance of successfully converting ventricular fibrillation to a regular heartbeat with defibrillation decreases by 10 percent with each passing minute. During the first minute of ventricular fibrillation, there is a 90 percent chance for successful conversion. If ventricular fibrillation persists for nine minutes, however, there is only a 10 percent chance for successful conversion with defibrillation. Therefore, the earlier defibrillation occurs, the better the patient's chance for survival.

2. *You are attempting resuscitation of a person in cardiac arrest. Because the patient is in a nonshockable form of cardiac arrest, the AED will not let you deliver a shock. How can you best provide care to this patient?*

   When an AED identifies nonshockable cardiac arrest, it will not let you deliver a shock. Nonshockable cardiac arrest is best treated with CPR and drugs given by advanced care providers. Therefore, the best treatment for a person in nonshockable cardiac arrest is continuous CPR and early advanced care.

3. *Of the following persons in shockable cardiac arrest, which stands the best chance for successful defibrillation with an AED? Why?*

   a. A person in cardiac arrest for one minute
   b. A person in cardiac arrest for five minutes
   c. A person in cardiac arrest for ten minutes

   The person in cardiac arrest for one minute stands the best chance for successful defibrillation. As stated in the first question, the chance of successfully converting ventricular fibrillation to a regular heartbeat by defibrillation decreases 10 percent with each passing minute. Therefore, the earlier defibrillation is administered, the better the patient's chance for survival.

REFERENCES

American Heart Association. (1997). *Basic life support for healthcare providers.* Dallas: Author.

Mistovitch, J., Benner, R., & Margolis, G. (1998). *Advanced cardiac life support.* Upper Saddle River, NJ: Prentice Hall/Brady.

CHAPTER

4

The Automated
External Defibrillator

LEARNING OBJECTIVES

At the end of this chapter, you will be able to

- Describe how the AED has simplified the process of defibrillation
- Identify and describe the basic components of the AED
- Describe the proper placement of the AED's electrodes on the patient's chest

---

KEY TERMS

Fully automated external defibrillator (FAED)—An AED that automatically analyzes the heart and delivers a defibrillating shock without any operator input.

Semiautomated external defibrillator (SAED)—An AED that requires the operator to manually activate the analysis and defibrillating shock when advised to do so by the AED.

Electrodes—Adhesive pads that attach to a cardiac arrest patient's chest and are connected by cables to an AED.

Data recording system—An audio or electronic component of an AED that permits documentation of a cardiac arrest incident while the AED is being used.

Early defibrillation can be a life-saving procedure for a person in cardiac arrest. A defibrillator is a device that delivers a defibrillating shock. An AED is a type of defibrillator that is attached to a patient's chest and automatically delivers an electrical shock to a heart in a shockable state of cardiac arrest. This chapter presents the AED and its basic components.

MANUAL DEFIBRILLATION AND A WEAK CHAIN OF SURVIVAL

Before AEDs, manual defibrillation was the only means of providing a defibrillating shock to a patient in cardiac arrest. Learning to provide manual defibrillation required extensive training. Consequently, few people were certified to perform this life-saving skill. Often, extended periods would pass before a person in cardiac arrest had access to defibrillation. Too frequently, by the time defibrillation could be administered, it was too late—the patient's condition had degenerated to a nonshockable state for which defibrillation held no benefit.

Thus before the AED, the weak link of early defibrillation created a weak Chain of Survival. The weak Chain of Survival resulted in poor survivability of cardiac arrest. In turn, cardiac arrest, especially when it occurred outside of a hospital, was considered a terminal event.

THE AED AND A STRONG CHAIN OF SURVIVAL

The automated external defibrillator has strengthened the weak link of early defibrillation. The AED is a small portable device capable of delivering a defibrillating shock. What makes the AED special is the way in which it simplifies the process of providing defibrillation.

When applied and activated, the AED automatically analyzes the heart in cardiac arrest and identifies it as either shockable or nonshockable. By doing so, the AED has reduced the extensive training requirements associated with manual defibrillation. Because the AED is portable, it can be brought to a patient's side, regardless of location—a definite advantage for those who suffer cardiac arrest outside of a hospital.

The less stringent instructional requirements mean that more people can be trained to provide emergency defibrillation. Training more people increases the access of defibrillation to those in need. Subsequently, defibrillation can be provided faster and on a more widespread basis. With defibrillation available sooner, the Chain of Survival is strong. The strong chain makes the chances of surviving cardiac arrest better than ever before!

TYPES OF AEDS

There are two types of AEDs. Although both types identify shockable and non-shockable forms of cardiac arrest, the procedures for operating them are slightly different.

Fully Automated External Defibrillators

Once turned on, a **fully automated external defibrillator (FAED)** analyzes the heart in cardiac arrest and decides whether it is in a shockable or nonshockable state. If the heart is shockable, the FAED warns the rescuers of a pending shock and then automatically delivers one to the patient's heart.

Semiautomated External Defibrillators

The **semiautomated external defibrillator (SAED)**, sometimes referred to as a **"shock advisory" defibrillator,** requires greater operator interaction in the process of heart analysis and defibrillation. After turning the AED on, the operator must press the ANALYZE button to allow the machine to analyze the heart of the person in cardiac arrest. If shockable cardiac arrest is identified, the SAED will advise the operator to defibrillate the person. Unlike the FAED, the SAED will not automatically defibrillate. Rather, the operator must press the SHOCK button to administer the defibrillating shock.

Although both types of AED are equally effective at identifying shockable and nonshockable cardiac arrest, the SAED is more popular because it is theoretically safer. An SAED will never deliver a defibrillation without the operator's authorization. As discussed later, rescuers must avoid all contact with patients during defibrillation. With an SAED, the operator can make sure all persons have cleared the patient before the shock is delivered.

The FAED is simpler to use than the SAED, however, because of the limited number of steps required for analysis and defibrillation. Once turned on, the machine does everything with minimal operator input. Because of the simplicity, FAEDs are useful for those with no medical knowledge.

Smart AEDs and Biphasic Defibrillation

Defibrillating shocks consist of electrical energy. Sometimes, shockable cardiac arrest can be converted to a normal heartbeat with a small amount of energy. Other times, larger quantities are required. It would seem to make sense, then, to administer a high level of electricity in all cases of shockable cardiac arrest.

Unfortunately, excessive electricity damages the heart, making resuscitation and long-term survival more difficult. Consequently, using the least amount of electricity that will effectively convert shockable cardiac arrest to a normal heartbeat is the best option.

Most AEDs deliver standard amounts of electricity that start low and increase with each shock if shockable cardiac arrest persists. However, there are new, **"smart" AEDs** that calculate the exact amount of electricity needed to successfully defibrillate a heart in shockable cardiac arrest (Mistovitch, Benner, & Margolis, 1998). Some new AEDs also use **biphasic defibrillation.** With biphasic defibrillation, the electrical current is reversed halfway through the shock. Studies have shown biphasic defibrillation to be more effective at converting shockable cardiac arrest while using lower levels of electricity.

AED COMPONENTS

Numerous companies manufacture AEDs. Despite the existence of different makes and models, all AEDs have several common components. The rescuer must be familiar with these components and their use in treating patients in cardiac arrest. Unfamiliarity creates confusion and can delay the early delivery of a defibrillating shock. Figure 4–1 shows a typical AED.

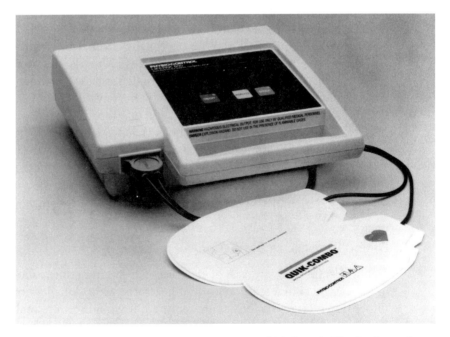

Figure 4–1   LIFEPAK 500/AED. Courtesy of Medtronic Physio-Control.

Control Panel

The body of the AED houses a control panel with buttons that control the operation of the AED. Generally, the control panel for an SAED contains three buttons:

ON/OFF: turns the AED on or off

ANALYZE: instructs the AED to analyze the heart of the person in cardiac arrest

SHOCK: delivers a defibrillating shock after the AED identifies a shockable state of cardiac arrest

FAEDs contain only the ON/OFF switch, as heart analysis and shock delivery are automatically performed by the device.

The number and layout of the buttons vary depending on the manufacturer and type of AED. A screen used for written communication (discussed later) is also located on the control panel.

Electrodes and Cables

Electrodes are large, self-adhesive pads that attach to the patient's chest. Two electrodes are needed. Cables connect the electrodes to the AED by way of a cable attachment port. Electrical signals from the heart are picked up by the electrodes and transmitted to the AED for analysis. By analyzing these electrical signals, the AED determines whether the heart is in a shockable or nonshockable state. If a shockable state of cardiac arrest is discovered, the AED will generate an electrical current and transmit it back through the cables to the electrodes. The electrodes then administer the defibrillating shock to the patient's heart.

The electrodes must be carefully placed on the patient's chest. One electrode is placed to the right of the sternum (breastbone), just below the collarbone. The second electrode is placed over the lower left ribs, just below the nipple (see Figure 4–2). Placing the electrodes in this manner directs electricity to the heart and allows for effective defibrillation.

On newer AEDs, the electrodes and cables are preconnected and packaged as one unit. However, some AEDs may require the operator to separately attach the cables and electrodes prior to use. Often, the cables are color coded and attached as follows:

White: attached to electrode right of the sternum

Red: attached to electrode over the lower left ribs

Most AEDs include illustrations or color-coded electrodes and/or cables to assist in proper placement (see Figure 4–1). Incorrect attachment may result in a failure to identify and defibrillate a shockable state.

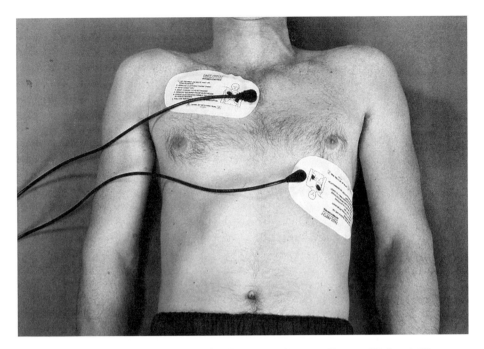

Figure 4–2   AED Electrode and Cable Placement (*Source:* Karren, Hafen, & Limmer, 1998, p. 144)

Note that some sources may discuss an alternative positioning of the electrodes. In the alternative position, the electrode with the white cable is placed on the front of the chest, over the top of the heart. The second electrode, with the red cable, is placed on the back, just under the left shoulder blade. *However, some AEDs will not function with the electrodes in this position!* Reference the manufacturer's guidelines for compatibility.

Electrodes are disposable and should be discarded after use. In addition, packaged electrodes have an expiration date, after which they must be replaced.

Batteries

Since it is a portable device, an AED requires batteries. Depending on the manufacturer, the batteries may be rechargeable or require total replacement when low. The batteries fit into the body of the AED and are easily removed when needed.

Low battery power is the number-one cause of AED malfunction! When batteries become low, they must immediately be replaced or recharged. Most AEDs conduct an internal battery check when turned on and will inform you of their status. All manufacturer guidelines concerning battery maintenance and replacement must be strictly followed. A fully charged spare set of batteries should be on hand at all times for emergency replacement. *The time to discover low batteries is before the AED is needed!*

Communication System

The **communication system** permits the AED to communicate with the rescuer. Depending on the manufacturer, different AEDs may have different types of communication systems. Synthesized voices that verbalize messages are standard on newer AEDs. Other forms of communication occur through lights or tones. Most AEDs have a screen for displaying text messages and graphics. Frequently AEDs have a communication system that incorporates all of these features.

The communication system is invaluable in prompting the rescuer during resuscitation of the patient. For example, the AED may instruct the operator to "perform one minute of CPR" or "press the SHOCK button to defibrillate." Additionally, the communication system may troubleshoot problems, such as low battery power or loose electrodes, or indicate when routine maintenance is required. Table 4–1 illustrates examples of verbal and written communication issued by AEDs.

Data Recording System

AEDs are equipped with different types of **data recording systems** that allow the operator to record information while simultaneously using the AED. Recording systems generally fall into two categories: voice and computer.

Table 4–1   Examples of Written or Verbal AED Messages

Procedure/Condition	*Example of Voice or Written Message*
Heart analysis	"Push analyze button now" "Analyzing now—stand clear!"
Shockable cardiac arrest identified	"Preparing to shock" "Push shock button now" "Shocking now—stand clear!"
Nonshockable state identified	"No shock advised" "Check pulse" "Heart is not shockable—check pulse"
Troubleshooting	"Batteries low" "Connect electrodes" "Electrodes are loose"

AEDs may have an audio recorder that permits the operator to verbally narrate and record the events of the entire cardiac arrest incident. The tape recorder must be activated and the following information verbalized:

- Date and time
- Patient and scene description
- All interventions, *as they occur*
- Patient response to all care (both positive and negative)

An internal computerized data storage system is the second type of recording system found in newer AEDs. Electrical heart rhythms, time of defibrillation, patient's response to defibrillation, and total number of defibrillations are just a few of the items that can be captured on a computerized recording system. Later, this information can be downloaded onto a computer and printed out. Such information is invaluable for research, education, and quality assurance purposes.

Other Features

AEDs may have additional accessories as well. Some AEDs can be plugged in to a manual defibrillator monitor, such as those carried by advanced care providers. Advanced care requires viewing the heart's electrical tracing, or **electrocardiogram (ECG)**, on the screen of a cardiac monitor. If the AED can be plugged in to such a monitor, then there's no need to replace the AED's electrodes and cables with the other device's. Some AEDs have a screen incorporated into their design just for this purpose.

This feature is also useful in treating nonshockable cardiac arrest. By viewing the heart's ECG, tailored drug therapy may be employed in an attempt to reverse the nonshockable state. Additionally, if a heartbeat is restored, the ensuing ECG can be evaluated, with additional care given as needed. Other accessories include a manual override device that permits defibrillation independent of the AED's decision not to shock.

OTHER EQUIPMENT NECESSARY FOR USE WITH AN AED

When providing emergency care with an AED, you will need additional equipment, including

- An extra set of fully charged batteries
- Two extra sets of electrodes

- A hand towel to dry wet or sweaty patients
- Scissors to remove clothing covering the chest
- An extra cassette tape for narration (if the AED contains an audio tape recorder)

This equipment should be kept with the AED at all times.

SAFETY AND EFFECTIVENESS OF THE AED

The AED has proven to be safe and effective at identifying shockable cardiac arrest and providing a defibrillating shock, and it has also been shown to be effective at identifying a nonshockable state and *withholding* a shock when necessary. When problems do occur, they are overwhelmingly attributable to human error, such as not replacing low batteries or improperly using the AED. *For the AED to be a life-saving tool, it must be maintained and used appropriately!*

SUMMARY

The AED has made the process of providing early defibrillation simpler. This simplification has allowed more people to complete training in emergency defibrillation. The greater the number of persons certified in defibrillation, the faster providers can reach the side of cardiac arrest patients. And the earlier defibrillation occurs, the more effective it is at converting a heart in a shockable state of cardiac arrest to one that can pump oxygen-rich blood to the body's cells and organs.

Remember that the AED is not necessarily a life-saving device by itself. For the AED to be effective, the remaining links in the Chain of Survival (early access, early CPR, early advanced care) must be strong. When the Chain of Survival is strong, surviving cardiac arrest is a distinct possibility.

FOOD FOR THOUGHT

To test your understanding, read and discuss the following questions.

1. *AEDs have made the delivery of emergency defibrillation easier than ever before. How has the AED accomplished this feat?*

   An AED automatically analyzes a heart in cardiac arrest and determines if it is in a shockable or nonshockable state. If the heart is in shockable cardiac arrest, it will advise the user to press the SHOCK button to administer a shock. FAEDs will automatically deliver a defibrillating shock without any operator input. If the patient is in a nonshockable state, the AED will not permit defibrillation to occur.

In the past, manual defibrillation required the provider to visually interpret the patient's ECG and decide whether defibrillation would be beneficial. This required many hours of training, and few people were certified to perform this task. By automatically analyzing hearts in cardiac arrest, AEDs have tremendously simplified the process of defibrillation and increased the numbers of people able to deliver the life-saving measure.

2. *You head a committee that is debating whether to buy an SAED or an FAED. What are the differences and similarities between these two types of AEDs?*

Although both types are equally effective at identifying shockable and non-shockable states of cardiac arrest and delivering a defibrillation when appropriate, they differ in the amount of operator input needed for analysis and defibrillation. FAEDs automatically analyze and deliver a defibrillating shock when shockable cardiac arrest is identified. SAEDs require the operator to physically press an ANALYZE and SHOCK button to analyze the cardiac arrest patient's heart and deliver a shock, respectively. SAEDs are more popular because they allow the operator to make sure that all persons have cleared away from the patient prior to defibrillation.

3. *Proper use of the AED requires specific placement of the electrodes on the chest of the person in cardiac arrest. Describe the appropriate placement of the electrodes.*

The electrodes of the AED must be carefully placed on the cardiac arrest patient's chest for maximum effectiveness. To correctly apply the two electrodes, place one to the right of the breastbone (sternum), just beneath the collarbone. Place the second electrode over the lower left ribs, just below the nipple. This positioning allows the AED to accurately analyze the heart in cardiac arrest and effectively defibrillate when needed.

4. *Maintaining fully charged batteries is essential for proper and effective use of the AED. Why?*

Since they are portable devices, AEDs require batteries. Fully charged batteries permit the AED to accurately analyze the cardiac arrest patient's heart and generate an effective electric current when needed. If the batteries are low, the AED may incorrectly identify shockable or nonshockable cardiac arrest or not function at all. As a result, a shockable form of cardiac arrest may go unshocked, or a nonshockable state may inappropriately receive a shock. In addition, low batteries pose a threat to the rescuer, since AED malfunction may result in provider injury.

REFERENCE

Karren, K. J., Hafen, B. Q., & Limmer, D. (1998). *First responder: A skills approach* (5th ed.) Upper Saddle River, NJ: Prentice Hall/Brady.

Mistovitch, J., Benner, R., & Margolis, G. (1998). *Advanced cardiac life support.* Upper Saddle River, NJ: Prentice Hall/Brady.

5

Patient Assessment

LEARNING OBJECTIVES

At the end of this chapter, you will be able to

- Describe the ABCs of patient assessment
- Identify the signs of cardiac arrest
- Describe the special procedures needed for a patient who may be suffering from a neck injury in addition to cardiac arrest
- Describe basic life support measures used to treat a cardiac arrest patient

---

KEY TERMS

Infectious disease—A disease that can cause infection of the rescuer.

Body substance isolation—Measures taken to limit the transmission of infectious diseases.

Patient assessment—A systematic evaluation of a patient's level of responsiveness, airway, breathing, and circulation. A patient assessment quickly reveals the presence or absence of cardiac arrest.

Traumatic neck injury—An injury to the neck that occurs when the cardiac arrest patient loses consciousness and falls, striking his or her head or neck.

Basic life support—Basic measures to support life. Basic life support includes opening the airway, performing rescue breathing, and performing CPR.

A group of patrons inform you, the security guard in a neighborhood park, that there is a man on the ground in the parking lot. After finding the man, they immediately came to the guard station to notify you. Quickly, you grab your AED and make the thirty-second trip to the parking lot. As you enter the lot, you notice several excited people frantically waving you over to the side of the groundskeeper, who is lying face down in the grass.

Is this patient in cardiac arrest?

To determine if a person is in cardiac arrest, you must assess them for the signs of unresponsiveness, breathlessness, and lack of a pulse. **Patient assessment** is a systematic evaluation that quickly enables you to determine whether these three signs of cardiac arrest are present. Since an AED should be applied only to persons in cardiac arrest, patient assessment is an important part of emergency cardiac care.

This chapter describes how to correctly assess a patient and identify cardiac arrest. In addition, it reviews **basic life support** for cardiac arrest patients.

INFECTIOUS DISEASES AND PERSONAL SAFETY

Before you learn about patient assessment, you must first know something about **infectious disease**. An infectious disease can be transmitted from a patient to a rescuer. Although the majority of infectious diseases do not present a threat to rescuers, there are a few that do have deadly consequences if transmitted. These include tuberculosis, hepatitis, meningitis, and human immunodeficiency virus (HIV).

For an infectious disease to be transmitted to a rescuer, fluids or substances from an infected patient must enter the rescuer's body. Body fluids or substances that can potentially transmit an infectious disease include blood, vomit, saliva, urine, feces, and amniotic fluid from an expectant mother. These body substances and fluids can get into a rescuer's body through his or her mouth, nose, or eyes or through an open wound.

More often than not, you will not know when a patient has an infectious disease. Many people with infectious diseases appear healthy and do not display signs of illness. Even if the presence of an infectious disease is obvious, it is impossible to determine which body fluids or substances are potentially dangerous. Consequently, the safest course of action is to assume that *all* patients have an infectious disease and *all* body substances are infectious, until proven otherwise.

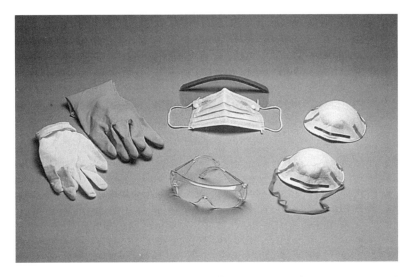

Figure 5–1   Examples of Body Substance Isolation Devices (*Source:* Bergeron & Bizjak, 1999, p. 23)

To decrease the chance of contracting an infectious disease, you must follow **body substance isolation (BSI)** guidelines. BSI guidelines are measures used to prevent rescuer contact with infectious fluids and substances. Medical gloves, goggles, masks, gowns, and barrier devices such as pocket masks and face shields are all examples of BSI devices (see Figure 5–1).

To properly assess a patient, you must physically touch him or her. Therefore, BSI precautions must be used on every patient. Gloves prevent entry of the patient's body fluids and substances through the rescuer's hands, and protective goggles prevent disease transmission through the rescuer's eyes. Pocket masks or face shields provide a barrier between you and the patient's mouth when delivering rescue breaths during CPR. Additionally, rescuers should wash their hands at the first possible moment after patient care has been terminated—*even if they wore gloves!*

HOW TO ASSESS A PATIENT

Scene Size-Up

Before physically touching a cardiac patient, you must first conduct a **scene size-up.** The scene size-up is a quick evaluation of the scene, during which you must ask yourself two basic questions: "Does the scene appear safe?" and "Has the patient suffered a neck injury?"

Scene Safety

Rescuer safety is the *number one* priority when delivering emergency cardiac care! Personal safety comes before patient assessment and even early defibrillation. The scene of a cardiac arrest can contain hazards that threaten the well-being of both the rescuers and the patient. Scene hazards can include a dangerous patient location, poor environmental conditions, and hostile bystanders or family members. As a rescuer, you cannot do any good if you are injured or placed in a threatening situation. Never enter a scene or deliver care unless it is safe to do so.

If a scene is or at any time becomes hazardous, either eliminate the cause or remove yourself from harm's way—even if such a move delays patient assessment and application of the AED. Depending on the type of hazard, resources like the police and fire department can help in establishing and maintaining a scene that is safe to deliver emergency cardiac care.

Traumatic Neck Injury

A **traumatic neck injury** is an injury caused by force or energy. Sometimes, traumatic injuries occur as a result of cardiac arrest. In cardiac arrest, many people fall as they lose consciousness. Frequently, a person who falls will strike his or her head, and any injury to the head may also cause injury to the spinal column, thus a neck injury. Since you cannot see a spinal injury in the neck, you must assume that any patient with an obvious injury (lacerations or bruising) to the head also

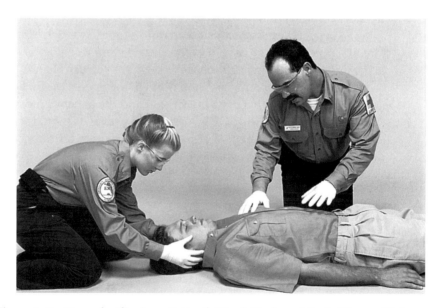

Figure 5–2   Properly Aligning a Patient's Head, Neck, and Back   (*Source:* Hafen, Karren, & Mistovich, 1996, p. 158)

has a traumatic neck injury. Quickly scan the patient for such injuries as you approach him or her.

Traumatic neck injuries require special care. If the spine or the neck has been injured, excessive movement of the patient's head or neck may cause permanent spinal damage, even if successful resuscitation occurs. To protect the spine in the neck, keep the head, neck, and back in a straight, neutral position, and prevent excessive head and neck movement (see Figure 5–2).

If you must move a person with a suspected neck injury, the head, neck, and back must be moved as a single unit.

The ABCs of Assessment

As discussed in Chapter One, the signs of cardiac arrest are unresponsiveness, breathlessness, and the lack of a pulse. To identify or rule out cardiac arrest, you must quickly determine whether or not these three signs are present.

If all three signs are present, the patient is in cardiac arrest. *If all three of these signs are not present, the patient is not in cardiac arrest!* Some medical emergencies produce a state of unresponsiveness accompanied by breathing and a pulse. Since these conditions do not represent cardiac arrest, application of the AED is inappropriate in such cases. An organized and thorough assessment will differentiate cardiac arrest from other conditions and result in appropriate use of the AED.

Note, however, that a patient may continue to breathe for several seconds following the onset of cardiac arrest. These respirations are gasping in nature, however, and do not represent normal breathing. Such breathing is short lived and will quickly progress to breathlessness. If gasping or shallow respirations are present without a pulse, assume that the patient is in cardiac arrest.

To assess a patient, perform the following steps, in the following order:

1. Determine unresponsiveness
2. Check the patient's airway
3. Check for breathing
4. Check for circulation (pulse)

The mnemonic *ABC* provides a simple way to remember the individual steps of patient assessment and the order in which to perform them: after determining unresponsiveness, check the patient's <u>A</u>irway, <u>B</u>reathing, and <u>C</u>irculation (pulse).

Step 1: Determine Unresponsiveness
An unresponsive patient is one who cannot be awakened. A person in cardiac arrest becomes unresponsive because his or her brain has been deprived of oxygen-rich

blood. For a patient without a neck injury, determine unresponsiveness by tapping or gently shaking the patient while shouting, "Can you hear me? Are you okay?" or "Open your eyes for me!" If the patient does not respond, he or she is unresponsive. If you believe that the patient has sustained a neck injury, do not shake him or her! Rather, hold the patient's head and neck still while tapping and shouting. Refer to Figure 5–2.

Not all unresponsive patients are in cardiac arrest! Many medical emergencies other than cardiac arrest can produce a state of unresponsiveness accompanied by breathing and a pulse. Therefore, continue the assessment instead of applying the AED.

If an unresponsive patient is in a confined or problematic area in which it is difficult to render further assessment and care, you will have to move the patient. Examples of such areas include rooftops, inside vehicles, or in small rooms such as bathrooms or hallways. In these cases, it may be necessary to move the patient to a location that affords a more workable environment. This task must be completed quickly, as a shockable state of cardiac arrest will quickly degenerate into a nonshockable form. If you suspect a neck injury, take care to move the patient's head, neck, and back as a single unit, as just described.

Step 2: Check the Airway

The airway provides a passageway through which air, and thus oxygen, is delivered into the lungs. Once in the lungs, oxygen is transferred to the blood, where it is circulated by the heart to the individual cells of the body. If the airway is blocked, or obstructed, oxygen will not pass into the lungs. Therefore, even during cardiac arrest, the airway must be kept open.

All unresponsive patients must have their airway opened and cleared if necessary. For the unresponsive patient without a neck injury, the airway is opened using the head tilt–chin lift maneuver. The head tilt–chin lift maneuver is best performed with the patient lying on his or her back (supine). If the patient is not in this position, roll him or her onto the back at this time.

The Head Tilt–Chin Lift Maneuver   See Figure 5–3 for an illustration of the **head tilt–chin lift maneuver.** To perform it, follow these steps:

1. Place a hand on the patient's forehead. With your other hand, place the tips of the fingers underneath the chin bone.
2. With one smooth motion, apply gentle backward pressure on the patient's forehead while simultaneously lifting the jaw upward with the fingertips.
3. Look inside the person's mouth and remove any visible obstructions such as loose dentures, food, or foreign objects.

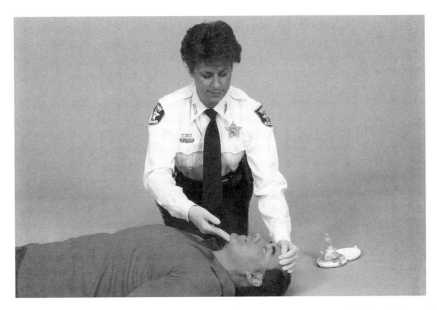

Figure 5–3   Head Tilt–Chin Lift Maneuver (*Source:* Bergeron & Bizjak, 1999, p. 85)

Because the head tilt–chin lift moves the head and neck, it should be avoided in cases where the patient has a suspected neck injury. Movement of the head and neck may worsen or cause permanent injury to the traumatically injured spine in the neck. Instead, the jaw-thrust maneuver should be used to open the airway.

Jaw-Thrust Maneuver   See Figure 5–4 for an illustration of the **jaw-thrust maneuver.** To perform it, follow these steps:

1. Kneel above the patient's head and place one forearm on each side of the patient's head.
2. Place your fingers, one hand to each side, on the bottom of the patient's jaw. Your thumbs should be placed on the patient's cheeks.
3. With a lifting motion, lift the patient's jaw upward.
4. Look inside the patient's mouth and remove any visible obstructions such as loose dentures, food, or foreign objects.

Like the head tilt–chin lift maneuver, the jaw-thrust maneuver is best performed with the patient on his or her back. When positioning the patient on his or her back, take care to move the head, neck, and back as a single unit.

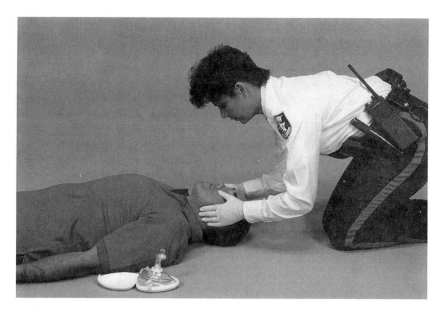

Figure 5–4   Jaw-Thrust Maneuver (*Source:* Bergeron & Bizjak, 1999, p. 85)

Once the airway has been opened and any obstructions removed, the head tilt–chin lift or jaw-thrust position should be maintained and the patient's breathing assessed.

Step 3: Check the Patient's Breathing

After opening and clearing the patient's airway, determine if the patient is breathing. A patient in a state of cardiac arrest will be breathless—that is, the patient will not be breathing. (As noted previously, however, a patient may continue to breath for several seconds after the onset of cardiac arrest. These respirations are gasping in nature and do not represent normal breathing. Such breathing is short lived and will quickly progress to breathlessness. If gasping or shallow respirations present without a pulse, assume that the patient is in cardiac arrest.) To determine whether or not the patient is breathing, place your ear near the patient's mouth and *look, listen,* and *feel* for breathing (see Figure 5–5).

Look at the patient's chest for the rise and fall associated with breathing. Simultaneously, listen and feel for air coming from the patient's mouth and nose. If the patient is breathless, chest movement and air passage through the mouth and nose will be absent.

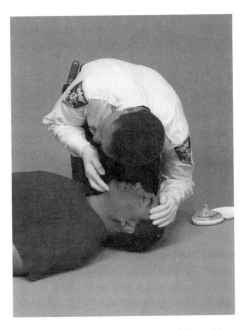

Figure 5–5   Looking, Listening, and Feeling for Breathing (*Source:* Bergeron & Bizjak, 1999, p. 88)

For a breathless patient, attempt two rescue breaths (see Appendix A). If possible, deliver rescue breaths using BSI barrier devices like pocket masks or face shields. All rescue breaths must be performed while holding the head tilt–chin lift or jaw-thrust maneuver to keep the airway open.

If the first rescue breath does not pass into the patient's lungs, reposition the head and attempt another one. Very possibly, the head tilt–chin lift maneuver did not adequately open the airway. If you used the jaw-thrust maneuver, relift the jaw. If the second rescue breath is unsuccessful, assume there is a foreign body airway obstruction, and attempt removal (see Appendix C).

Although breathlessness should increase your suspicion of cardiac arrest, not all breathless patients are necessarily in cardiac arrest. Some medical conditions may cause breathlessness before causing cardiac arrest. Therefore, assessing the patient's circulation is necessary before determining if he or she is in cardiac arrest.

Step 4: *Checking the Patient's Circulation (Pulse)*
This step determines whether or not the patient has a pulse. A pulse is produced when blood pumped by the heart surges through the arteries. Where the arteries

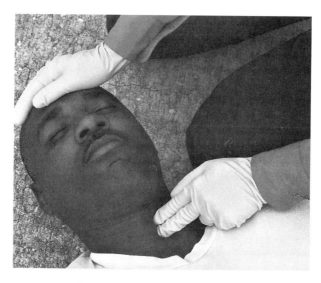

Figure 5–6   Locating the Carotid Pulse (*Source:* Bergeron & Bizjak, 1999, p. 135)

lie close to the body's surface, a pulse is felt. In cardiac arrest, blood is not circulated, and so the patient lacks a pulse.

The **carotid artery** is the most reliable site for determining the presence or absence of a pulse. To locate the carotid pulse, find the patient's larynx (Adam's apple or voice box). Gently lay your index and middle fingers on top of the Adam's apple and slide them toward you into the groove located on the side of the patient's neck. If present, the carotid pulse will be felt within this groove (see Figure 5–6). Assessing for a pulse should take five to ten seconds.

If your assessment shows the patient to be unresponsive, breathless, and lacking a pulse, the patient is in cardiac arrest! Once cardiac arrest has been identified, placement of the AED must immediately follow. If several rescuers are present, CPR should be initiated while the AED is prepared. If you have an AED and are by yourself, do not start CPR but prepare and apply the AED. In this situation, the benefits of early defibrillation outweigh those of CPR. If an AED is not yet available, perform CPR until a defibrillator arrives and is ready for use (see Appendix B). Overall care of the cardiac arrest patient with an AED is discussed in Chapter Six.

CARE FOR PATIENTS NOT IN CARDIAC ARREST

If the patient is not in cardiac arrest, do not apply an AED! Following are some of the ways patients not in cardiac arrest can present.

Responsive, Breathing, and with a Pulse

For a patient who is responsive, is breathing, and has a pulse, turn your attention to providing comfort measures and emotional support. If available, medical oxygen delivered through an oxygen mask is beneficial.

Unresponsive, Breathing, and with a Pulse

If an unresponsive patient is adequately breathing and there is no evidence of a neck injury, place the patient in the recovery position. To do so, place the patient on his or her side to keep the airway open. Should the patient vomit, this position allows the vomit and other secretions to drain from the mouth instead of into the throat, where they can cause an airway occlusion. See Figure 5–7 for an illustration of the recovery position.

If you suspect a neck injury, do not place the patient in the recovery position. Moving the patient into the recovery position unduly moves the head, neck, and back and may cause permanent damage. Rather, maintain the jaw-thrust position until advanced care arrives. If the patient vomits, turn the patient onto his or her side, moving the head, neck, and back as a single unit.

If the person's breathing is inadequate, perform rescue breathing. The use of a pocket mask or face shield is recommended. If available, medical oxygen should be delivered simultaneously.

Unresponsive and Breathless but with a Pulse

The unresponsive patient who is breathless but has a pulse is said to be suffering respiratory arrest. If breathing is not resumed, the lack of oxygen intake will cause rapid progression to cardiac arrest. Therefore, the immediate delivery of rescue breaths is important. As discussed previously, barrier devices should

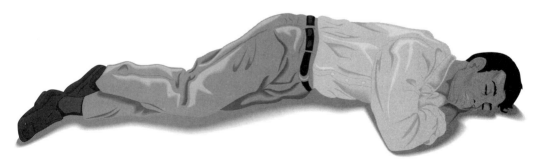

Figure 5–7   The Recovery Position (*Source:* Karren, Hafen, & Limmer, 1998, p. 92)

be used in delivering rescue breathing. If medical oxygen is available, it should be administered simultaneously.

Unresponsive with a Pulse and a Foreign Body Airway Obstruction

For the unresponsive patient with a foreign body obstructing the airway, immediate removal is necessary to prevent cardiac arrest. See Appendix C for recommendations on removing a foreign body from the airway.

CASE STUDY SUMMARY

As you approach the groundskeeper, you responsibly apply BSI protection in the form of gloves and protective eyewear. Quick observation reveals a male patient lying face down in the grass. The scene appears safe, so you inquire if anyone saw what occurred. A man steps forward and states that the patient was carrying some weeds when he suddenly collapsed. You instruct the man to call 911 and request an advanced care ambulance for a possible cardiac arrest.

Looking at the patient, you notice some blood coming from a small cut on the side of the patient's face. Realizing that he probably hit his head on collapse, you elect to observe all precautions in association with a possible traumatic neck injury. While holding his head still, you tap the man and shout "Can you hear me? Are you okay?" Since the patient does not respond, you realize that he is unresponsive. The man who telephoned for the ambulance returns and asks whether he can be of any help. You welcome his invitation and throw him a set of medical exam gloves.

Because the man is face down in the grass, you cannot properly assess his airway. With the help of the bystander, you carefully turn the patient over, with special attention to moving the patient's head, neck, and back as a single unit.

Once the patient is on his back, you perform a jaw-thrust maneuver to open the airway. You look inside his mouth and do not see any obstructions. After assessing the airway, you turn your attention toward his breathing. While maintaining the jaw-thrust position, you place your face

---

In Cardiac Arrest and with a Full Airway Obstruction

If a patient in cardiac arrest has a full airway obstruction, removal of the foreign body must *precede* application of the AED. Although this delays defibrillation, there is little chance of resuscitating a person in cardiac arrest if oxygen cannot be delivered to the cells of the heart, even when a shockable state exists. Therefore, the airway must be cleared and open. Once the airway has been cleared, the AED can then be applied and used. Again, see Appendix C for recommendations on removing a foreign body from the airway.

over the top of the patient's face and turn your view toward the patient's chest.

You do not see the chest rise and fall, as would be seen with an individual who is breathing. Additionally, you do not hear or feel any air movement at the patient's mouth and nose. You recognize that the patient is not breathing. You reach for your pocket mask, apply it to the patient's face, and deliver one rescue breath. The rescue breath passes easily into the patient's lungs, and the patient's chest rises in response. You deliver a second rescue breath, identical to the first.

Knowing that you must evaluate the patient's pulse, you instruct your helper to take over maintaining the jaw-thrust position and to begin administering rescue breathing. The young man takes over the jaw-thrust position and states that he thinks the head should be extended backward so as to allow a clearer passage for air into the lungs. You quickly inform him that since the patient fell and hit his head after becoming unresponsive, he may have a neck injury. Therefore, no undue movement of the head and neck should occur, for fear of causing permanent damage to the fragile spine. He obliges and delivers rescue breaths with another pocket mask you have provided.

With the patient's head stabilized, his airway open, and rescue breaths being delivered, you quickly feel for a carotid pulse. After five seconds you cannot locate a pulse and determine that the patient is unresponsive, breathless, and lacking a pulse. Realizing that the patient is in cardiac arrest, you ask the helper if he knows CPR. He states that he does and proceeds to perform one-person CPR while you ready the AED for application.

In cases where the patient is not in cardiac arrest, you must be physically and mentally prepared for the sudden onset of cardiac arrest. Additionally, even though the patient is not in cardiac arrest, advanced care must be notified for further treatment.

SUMMARY

Patient assessment is a systematic examination that permits you to quickly determine if a patient is in cardiac arrest. Because the AED is only used in cases of cardiac arrest, the patient assessment will determine when to apply the AED.

Since time is of the essence, patient assessment must be quick yet thorough. The rescuer cannot afford to overlook critical findings that may misdirect care or delay application of the AED. A sloppy assessment can cause a shockable patient to go unshocked or allow a patient with a pulse to receive defibrillation. Consequently, patient assessment is a critical part of emergency cardiac care.

FOOD FOR THOUGHT

To test your understanding, read and discuss the following questions.

1. *You have determined that a forty-two-year-old male is in cardiac arrest. Family members inform you that the patient has HIV. How will you handle this situation?*

   HIV is an infectious disease that can be transferred to the rescuer if he or she is not careful. To avoid transfer, the rescuer should use gloves, goggles, and pocket mask for protection. Additionally, any exposed wounds that the rescuer may have should be covered, and hand washing must immediately follow the resuscitation. Avoid contact with any and all obvious body fluids and substances. Many infectious diseases, including HIV, do not outwardly present with obvious signs and symptoms. Therefore, body substance isolation measures should be taken for every patient encounter.

2. *A person in cardiac arrest has fallen from a standing position and struck his head, as evidenced by a large laceration on his forehead. What special precautions must you take when delivering emergency care to this person?*

   A traumatic injury to the head may also cause an injury to the neck. If you see a fresh cut or someone witnesses the patient striking his or her head during a fall, suspect a possible traumatic neck injury. If the spine in the neck is injured, undue movement can cause permanent damage, even if a successful resuscitation occurs. To avoid causing permanent spinal damage, observe these precautions:

- Hold the head, neck, and back still when assessing for unresponsiveness
- Do not shake the patient when assessing for unresponsiveness
- Use the jaw-thrust maneuver instead of the head tilt–chin lift maneuver

Since you cannot see a spinal injury in the neck, assume that any patient with an obvious injury to the head also has an injured spine!

3. *You find an unresponsive female patient at her dining table. You perform a head tilt–chin lift maneuver to open her airway. Assessment of her breathing reveals the patient to be breathless. Your first rescue breath does not pass through to the lungs. Accordingly, you reposition the head and attempt a second rescue breath. Like the first, the second rescue breath does not pass. What must you do?*

If the patient is breathless and two rescue breaths do not pass through to the lungs, you must suspect a foreign body airway obstruction. A foreign body obstruction blocks the airway and will not let oxygen pass into the body during rescue breathing. Without oxygen, the cells of the body will die. For this reason, a foreign body airway obstruction must be cleared before you finish the assessment and use the AED if needed—even if the person is in cardiac arrest. Refer to Appendix C for recommendations on clearing a foreign body airway obstruction. After the foreign body is cleared from the airway and two rescue breaths can be delivered with ease, continue assessing the patient by checking the pulse, and apply the AED if needed.

4. *You are responding to a possible cardiac arrest with a new team member (CPR certified) who is scheduled to take a certified AED course in one week. The rookie asks you what patient assessment is and why it is so important. How would you respond?*

Patient assessment is a systematic evaluation that enables you to quickly identify whether a patient is in cardiac arrest. By examining the patient's level of consciousness, airway, breathing, and circulation, you can quickly determine if the patient is unresponsive, breathless, and lacking a pulse. Since the AED is only applied in instances of cardiac arrest, patient assessment is an important part of emergency cardiac resuscitation.

REFERENCES

Bergeron, J. D., & Bizjak, G. (1999). *First responder* (5th ed.). Upper Saddle River, NJ: Prentice Hall.

Hafen, B. Q., Karren, K. J., & Mistovich, J. J. (1996). *Prehospital emergency care* (5th ed.). Upper Saddle River, NJ: Prentice Hall.

Karren, K. J., Hafen, B. Q., & Limmer, D. (1998). *First responder: A skills approach* (5th ed.) Upper Saddle River, NJ: Prentice Hall/Brady.

6

Cardiac Arrest Resuscitation with the AED

LEARNING OBJECTIVES

At the end of this chapter, you will be able to

- Describe the sequence of patient assessment, CPR, and AED operation when resuscitating a person in cardiac arrest
- Identify the operational difference between an FAED and an SAED
- Describe how to provide emergency care when a "NO SHOCK" message is received
- Describe the emergency care needed when defibrillation successfully restores a heartbeat

---

KEY TERMS

Analysis—The process by which an AED evaluates a cardiac arrest patient's heart and decides whether the heart is shockable or nonshockable.

"SHOCK" message—The message displayed by an AED that has determined that a heart in cardiac arrest is in a shockable state and will benefit from a defibrillating shock.

"NO SHOCK" message—The message displayed by an AED that has determined that a heart in cardiac arrest is in a nonshockable state and will not benefit from a defibrillating shock.

Stacked shocks—A set of up to three shocks delivered consecutively by an AED as long as the heart is in a shockable state.

This year, your county has become progressive in how it provides emergency cardiac care. After considerable planning, an AED and a cardiac rescue team have been placed at this summer's county fair. Because of your pivotal role in the project, you have been appointed leader of a three-member rescue team. Each team member has been certified in CPR and use of the AED.

During the second night of the fair, your portable radio suddenly crackles with the voice of an excited vendor who states that he has just witnessed a man collapse near the rodeo grounds. You realize that this may be the case where you actually save a life. Quickly, you and your team board the specially equipped pickup with the SAED in hand. As you race to the scene, you instruct the local 911 center to send an advanced care ambulance to the location. Mentally, you review the steps of patient assessment and cardiac arrest resuscitation. By the stern look on your team's faces, you realize that they are doing the same. Everyone has applied gloves and protective face and eyewear.

Once at the rodeo grounds, you see a panicked crowd waving you to a fifty-six-year-old man lying on his back in the grass. On approach, you ensure that the scene is safe, and quickly scan the patient for signs of traumatic neck injury. Finding no such signs, you instruct one team member to perform the patient assessment. She declares the man to be unresponsive, breathless, and without a pulse. "The patient is in cardiac arrest!" she states.

How would you proceed?

Cardiac arrest resuscitation is the process of delivering emergency care to a cardiac arrest patient. Restoring a heartbeat to a heart that has stopped pumping blood is the goal of cardiac arrest resuscitation. As discussed in Chapter Two, resuscitation does not consist solely of early defibrillation. Rather, the AED must be used in conjunction with patient assessment and the four links in the Chain of Survival. Moreover, if resuscitation is to be successful, it must be delivered in a smooth and organized manner.

This chapter discusses operation of the AED in combination with patient assessment and CPR, to illustrate the most effective way to provide emergency care to a person in cardiac arrest.

GENERAL PRINCIPLES GUIDING THE USE OF AEDs

When you use an AED, you must remember eight general principles. When followed, these principles enable you to use an AED in a safe and effective manner.

1. *Locate the AED to the* left *side of the patient's head.* When the AED is placed next to the patient's left ear, the AED and its operator are in easy view of all team members. Placement of the electrodes is simpler from the left side of the patient, and CPR can easily be supervised by the operator if performed from the right side (American Heart Association, 1998). Unfortunately, this layout is not possible in every cardiac arrest situation; therefore, all rescuers must be adaptable to alternative positioning when required.

2. *Apply an AED only to a patient who is in cardiac arrest.* As discussed previously, a person in cardiac arrest is unresponsive, breathless, and without a pulse. If all three signs are not present, the patient is not in cardiac arrest, and the AED must not be applied.

   Attaching an AED to a person not in cardiac arrest leaves open the possibility, albeit slight, of administering an inadvertent shock. An inadvertent shock may cause injury or death, not only to the patient but also to the rescuer.

   An exception to this rule pertains to the cardiac arrest patient for whom early defibrillation has restored a heartbeat. Since the probability of lapsing back into cardiac arrest is significant, it is appropriate to leave the AED attached.

3. *Never delay defibrillation.* Never delay applying an AED to a person in cardiac arrest. Remember that successful defibrillation occurs early! As a general rule, you should strive to perform defibrillation within sixty seconds of the AED's arriving at the patient's side. However, it is recognized that in some situations this may not be possible, such as when a cardiac arrest patient must be moved from a dangerous situation.

   If you have an AED but no one to help you, do not delay applying the AED by initiating CPR. The benefits of early defibrillation outweigh those of CPR. Similarly, if an AED is nearby, it is allowable to leave the patient to retrieve it. If two or more rescuers are present, one should prepare the AED while the other(s) perform CPR.

4. *Never touch the patient or the AED while the AED is analyzing the patient's heart.* When an AED is analyzing a patient's heart, neither the AED nor the patient can be touched. Touching or moving the patient may interfere with the AED's ability to accurately identify a shockable or nonshockable state. It is the responsibility of the AED operator to make sure that all rescuers are clear of the patient and that CPR has been stopped.

5. *Never touch the patient during defibrillation.* Defibrillation involves the delivery of electricity to the heart. Although this electricity may be beneficial for a heart in cardiac arrest, it is not beneficial for a normally beating heart! Physically touching the patient can transfer the electrical shock to the rescuer. As a result, the rescuer may suffer injury or even cardiac arrest. An SAED allows the operator to clear all rescuers from the patient prior to pressing the SHOCK button. Before defibrillating, the operator verbally clears all rescuers by loudly stating, "Everybody clear the patient!" as well as making eye contact to ensure that everyone has complied with the order.

6. *Notify advanced care early.* As discussed previously, early defibrillation does not replace the need for advanced care. Advanced care provides important medical attention for the patient who has been successfully defibrillated or is in a nonshockable state of cardiac arrest. Request advanced care as early as possible. If advanced care is not available, the patient must be transported to a medical facility capable of providing advanced care.

7. *Avoid radio interference.* Radio transmissions may interfere with an AED's ability to accurately analyze a heart. Although newer AEDs account for this interference, it is suggested that all radio usage take place at least six feet from the defibrillator during **analysis**. Consult the individual manufacturer recommendations for specific guidelines concerning radio interference.

8. *Remember that AEDs deliver "stacked shocks."* AEDs deliver defibrillating shocks in individual sets each consisting of up to three consecutive shocks (delivered one right after another). After one set of **stacked shocks** (three sequential shocks) has been delivered, one minute of CPR is performed, as discussed later in this chapter.

   An AED will continue to deliver stacked shocks as long as a shockable form of cardiac arrest is present. Once a heart becomes nonshockable, however, the AED will no longer deliver shocks, *even if an entire sequence of three shocks has not been completed.* For example, if after one shock the heart enters a nonshockable state, the AED will not deliver the second and third shocks. Likewise, for the patient who enters a nonshockable state after the second shock, the AED will not administer a third shock. If the patient's heart remains shockable after one full set of three stacked shocks, the rescuer performs one minute of CPR before the AED performs another analysis and delivers a second set of up to three stacked shocks.

Resuscitation of a Cardiac Arrest Patient with an AED

The best emergency cardiac care is systematic and organized. After ensuring everyone's personal safety and quickly scanning for signs of a neck injury, the rescuer determines patient unresponsiveness and performs the ABCs of assessment. If the patient is in cardiac arrest, the rescuer must quickly apply the AED. If the AED identifies a shockable form of cardiac arrest, the rescuer performs the following sequence of actions:

1. Deliver up to three stacked shocks.
2. Check pulse and administer one minute of CPR (if still in cardiac arrest).
3. Reanalyze the heart.
4. Repeat above steps until a pulse is found or the AED delivers a "NO SHOCK" message.

If at anytime a pulse is found or the AED issues a "NO SHOCK" message, the care provided will change. These changes are described later in the chapter.

Keep in mind that operational differences exist between SAEDs and FAEDs. Additionally, variances occur when one rescuer as opposed to several provides emergency care. Where applicable, these differences are noted.

Step-by-Step Procedures for Using an AED

The following paragraphs provide a step-by-step discussion of how to resuscitate a cardiac arrest patient using an AED.

1. *Prepare yourself mentally and physically.* While moving to the patient's location, mentally review the steps of patient assessment, the signs of cardiac arrest, and the procedure of resuscitating a patient with an AED. Apply BSI items like gloves and protective face and eyewear. Additionally, ensure that an AED is readily handy, or follow predetermined measures for obtaining one. Request advanced care assistance.
2. *Size up the scene.* Make sure the scene is safe and free of hazards. Quickly look for evidence of neck injury as you approach the patient. If you suspect traumatic neck injury, take the special neck injury precautions described in Chapter Five.
3. *Assess the patient and provide basic care.* Assess the patient to determine if he or she is in cardiac arrest (check for unresponsiveness and then check the patient's airway, breathing, and circulation). (See Figure 6–1 for an illustration.) If bystanders or other rescuers have initiated CPR, instruct them to stop while you assess the patient. If you suspect the patient has a neck injury, take the necessary precautions when positioning the patient and opening his or her airway. If the patient is breathless, deliver two rescue breaths. If the patient is without a pulse, have another rescuer or bystander start CPR. If the patient is *not* in cardiac arrest, continue care as discussed later in the chapter.

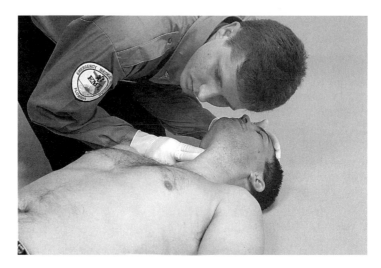

Figure 6–1   Patient Assessment (*Source:* Hafen, Karren, & Mistovich, 1996, p. 317)

4. *Turn on the AED and apply the electrodes.* Place the AED to the left of the patient's head and turn it on. Attach the AED's electrodes and cables to the patient's chest as described in Chapter Four. If the AED has a recorder for narration, begin narration while simultaneously applying the electrodes.

   As noted previously, the AED operator must never delay preparing the AED to assist with CPR! This will only delay early defibrillation. Even

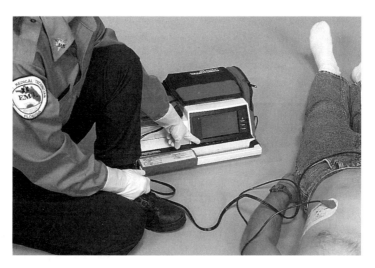

Figure 6–2   Turning on the AED and Applying the Electrodes (*Source:* Hafen, Karren, & Mistovich, 1996, p. 317)

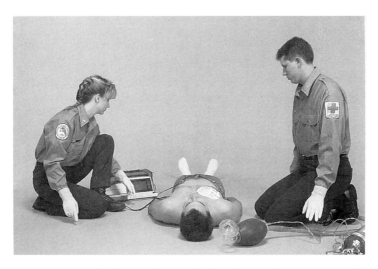

Figure 6–3   Analyzing the Heart (*Source:* Hafen, Karren, & Mistovich, 1996, p. 317)

when acting alone, do not initiate CPR, but prepare the AED for use. Immediate defibrillation outweighs the benefits of CPR. (Figure 6–2 illustrates this step.)

5. *Analyze the heart.* Stop CPR and clear all rescuers from the patient by stating, "Everybody clear the patient!" (See Figure 6–3 for an illustration.) Press the ANALYZE button. (FAEDs will begin analysis without operator activation.) When the AED is finished analyzing the patient's heart, it will issue a "SHOCK" or "NO SHOCK" message.
   - *If you get a "SHOCK" message,* the AED has identified a shockable form of cardiac arrest that must immediately be defibrillated. Proceed to Step 6.
   - *If you get a "NO SHOCK" message,* the heart is in a nonshockable state and cannot be shocked. Refer to the section later in the chapter on continued care following a "NO SHOCK" message.

6. *Deliver a shock.* Clear all rescuers from the patient by stating, "Everybody clear the patient!" Establish eye contact with all rescuers to ensure that all are clear. Press the SHOCK button to deliver the first shock. An FAED will automatically deliver the first shock, after giving a warning. (Figure 6–4 illustrates this step.)

7. *Reanalyze the heart.* Do not check for a pulse, but immediately press the ANALYZE button to reanalyze the patient's heart. You must determine if the heart is still shockable, if it has converted to nonshockable cardiac arrest, or if it has regained a heart beat. (All FAEDs and some SAEDs will automatically reanalyze the heart without any operator input.) When the AED is finished analyzing the patient's heart, it will display a "SHOCK" or "NO SHOCK" message:

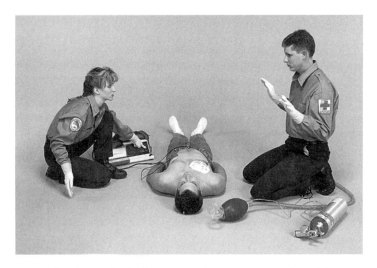

Figure 6–4   Delivering a Shock (*Source:* Hafen, Karren, & Mistovich, 1996, p. 317)

- *If you get a "SHOCK" message,* the AED has identified a shockable form of cardiac arrest that must immediately be defibrillated. Deliver a second defibrillating shock as described in Step 8.
- *If you get a "NO SHOCK" message,* the AED has identified a nonshockable form of cardiac arrest, or the patient has regained a heartbeat. Refer to the section later in this chapter on continued care following a "NO SHOCK" message.

8. *Deliver a second shock.* Since the AED has identified a shockable form of cardiac arrest, deliver a second shock, following the procedure in Step 6.

9. *Again reanalyze the heart.* Immediately reanalyze the patient's heart, as discussed in Step 7. The AED will again give a "SHOCK" or "NO SHOCK" message:
   - *If you get a "SHOCK" message,* the AED has identified a shockable form of cardiac arrest that must immediately be defibrillated. Deliver a third shock, as described in Step 10.
   - *If you get a "NO SHOCK" message,* the AED has identified a nonshockable form of cardiac arrest, or the patient has regained a heartbeat. Refer to the section later in this chapter on continued care following a "NO SHOCK" message.

10. *Deliver a third shock.* Since the AED has identified shockable cardiac arrest, deliver a third defibrillating shock, following the procedure in Step 6.

    At this point, a total of three shocks have been given. Together, these three shocks constitute one complete set of three stacked shocks. After you have delivered a complete set of stacked shocks, you must put further

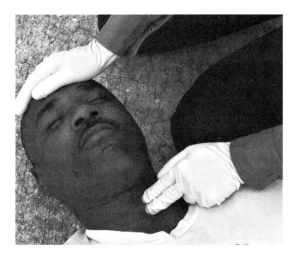

Figure 6–5   Checking for a Pulse (*Source:* Bergeron & Bizjak, 1999, p. 135)

analysis and defibrillation on hold temporarily. Instead, you must check for a pulse and perform one minute of CPR if needed. For the time being, preserving the cells of the heart, brain, and other organs with oxygen-rich blood outweighs further defibrillation.

11. *Check for a pulse.* Check for a carotid pulse as described in Chapter Five (see Figure 6–5).
    - *If a pulse is present,* proceed to the section later in this chapter on continued care when a pulse is found.
    - *If no pulse is present,* state, "No pulse present. The patient is still in cardiac arrest!" and continue with Step 12.

12. *Perform one minute of CPR.* If the patient does not have a pulse, perform CPR for one minute (see Figure 6–6). *Do not remove the AED from the patient!* See Appendix B for guidelines concerning CPR.

13. *Again reanalyze the heart.* After one minute of CPR, reanalyze the patient's heart as described in Step 7. When the AED is finished analyzing the patient's heart, a "SHOCK" message or "NO SHOCK" message will be given:
    - *If you get a "SHOCK" message,* the AED has identified a shockable form of cardiac arrest that must immediately be defibrillated. Begin delivery of a second set of up to three stacked shocks as described in Step 14.
    - *If you get a "NO SHOCK" message,* the AED has identified a nonshockable form of cardiac arrest, or the patient has regained a heartbeat. Refer to the section later in this chapter on continued care following a "NO SHOCK" message.

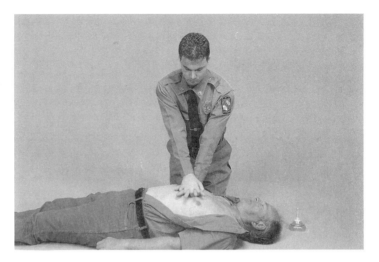

Figure 6–6   Performing CPR (*Source:* Bergeron & Bizjak, 1999, p. 172)

14. *Deliver a second set of stacked shocks.* Since the AED has identified a shock-able form of cardiac arrest, deliver a fourth defibrillating shock, following the procedure in Step 6. Then immediately reanalyze the patient's heart as described in Step 7.

    As long as the AED continues to identify shockable cardiac arrest, deliver a second set of up to three stacked shocks with reanalysis occurring between the fourth and fifth and the fifth and sixth shocks.

    Do not check for a pulse after the fourth and fifth shock, as this may cause the AED to inaccurately identify a shockable or nonshockable state of the heart or delay further shocks. If at anytime the AED delivers a "NO SHOCK" message, proceed to the section later in this chapter on continued care following a "NO SHOCK" message. If you end up delivering another complete set of three stacked shocks, continue with Step 15.

15. *Check for a pulse.* After delivering a second set of three stacked shocks, check for a carotid pulse.
    • *If a pulse is present,* proceed to the section later in this chapter on con-tinued care when a pulse is found.
    • *If no pulse is present,* state, "No pulse present. The patient is still in car-diac arrest!" and continue with Step 16.

16. *Perform one minute of CPR.* If the patient does not have a pulse, perform CPR for one minute. *Do not remove the AED from the patient!* See Appen-dix B for guidelines concerning CPR.

17. *Reanalyze the heart and perform further defibrillations as needed.* After one minute of CPR, reanalyze the patient's heart with the AED. Follow the technique as described in Step 7.

If the heart remains shockable, deliver another set of up to three stacked shocks as described in Step 14. If at any time the AED delivers a "NO SHOCK" message, follow the procedures described later in the chapter for continued care following a "NO SHOCK" message. If you end up delivering a third set of three stacked shocks, proceed to Step 18.

18. *Check for a pulse.* After delivering a third set of three stacked shocks, check for a carotid pulse.
    - *If a pulse is present,* proceed to the section later in this chapter on continued care when a pulse is found.
    - *If no pulse is present,* state, "No pulse present. The patient is still in cardiac arrest!" Perform one minute of CPR and then reanalyze the patient's heart as described in Step 17.

    Then repeat Steps 17 through 18 until one of the following occurs:
    a. A pulse is felt. Refer to the section later in this chapter on continued care when a pulse is felt.
    b. The AED returns a "NO SHOCK" message. Refer to the section later in this chapter on continued care following a "NO SHOCK" message.
    c. You turn care over to advanced care personnel.

Continued Care When a Pulse Is Found

If the patient has a pulse, immediately check for breathing. If the patient is adequately breathing, provide medical oxygen through a face mask, if available. In the absence of a traumatic neck injury, place the patient in the recovery position. If you suspect a traumatic neck injury, do not place the patient in the recovery position but maintain the jaw-thrust position until advanced care arrives. If the patient vomits, move the head, neck, and back as a single unit and turn the patient onto his or her side. Reperform the patient assessment every thirty seconds. If the patient falls back into cardiac arrest, use the AED as described previously.

If the patient is not breathing or barely breathing, initiate rescue breathing. See Appendix A for guidelines concerning rescue breathing. If available, medical oxygen should be delivered simultaneously. As before, reperform the patient assessment every thirty seconds. If the patient falls back into cardiac arrest, proceed as described previously.

Continued Care Following a "NO SHOCK" Message

If the AED gives a "NO SHOCK" message, the patient has either regained a heartbeat or developed a nonshockable form of cardiac arrest. When a "NO SHOCK" message is received, check for a carotid pulse. If a pulse is felt, the patient has been successfully converted from cardiac arrest and should be treated as just described in the section on continued care when a pulse is found.

If a pulse is *not* felt, the patient is in nonshockable cardiac arrest. State, "No pulse present. The patient is still in cardiac arrest!" and continue with the following care:

1. *Perform CPR for one minute.* With defibrillation no longer an option, oxygen-rich blood must be artificially circulated to preserve the body cells and organs. See Appendix B for recommendations concerning CPR.
2. *Analyze the heart.* Stop CPR after one minute and press the ANALYZE button to reanalyze the heart. Make sure all rescuers are clear of the patient.
   - *If the AED displays a "SHOCK" message,* the heart has returned to a shockable state. Prepare for defibrillation by clearing all rescuers from the patient. Proceed as described previously (Step 6 of the step-by-step instructions) and continue care from that point.
   - *If the AED displays a "NO SHOCK" message,* check for a carotid pulse.

If you feel a pulse, the patient has been successfully converted from cardiac arrest and should be treated as described previously in the section on continued care after a pulse is found. If you do *not* feel a pulse, the patient remains in nonshockable cardiac arrest. Perform one minute of CPR and then reanalyze the heart. Continue the sequence of CPR (one minute) followed by analysis with the AED until a state of shockable cardiac arrest returns, a pulse is found, or three consecutive "NO SHOCK" messages are received (United States Department of Transportation, 1994).

If after three consecutive *"NO SHOCK"* messages the patient remains without a pulse, extend the period of CPR to between one and two minutes. At this point the patient will have been in a nonshockable state of cardiac arrest for some time, and a return to a shockable state is extremely unlikely. For this reason, analysis with the AED can be performed at less frequent intervals. If at any time shockable cardiac arrest returns, immediately defibrillate as described previously (Step 6).

Procedures Once Advanced Care Arrives

Once advanced care arrives, the operator of the AED must give a brief report to the advanced care giver. The following information should be conveyed:

- Results of the initial patient assessment
- Results of the AED's analysis
- Number of shocks delivered, if applicable, and patient response
- Continued care given and present status of the patient

CASE STUDY SUMMARY

Once at the rodeo grounds, you see a panicked crowd waving you to a fifty-six-year-old man lying on his back in the grass. On approach, you ensure that the scene is safe, and you quickly scan for signs of traumatic neck injury. Finding no such signs, you instruct one team member to perform the patient assessment. She declares the man to be unresponsive, breathless, and without a pulse. "The patient is in cardiac arrest!" she states.

The two members of your team begin CPR as you prepare the AED for application. Once the AED is ready, CPR is stopped and you turn the AED on and quickly place the electrodes on the patient's chest. Once these are in place, you press the ANALYZE button, after ensuring that all rescuers and bystanders are clear of the patient. Simultaneously, you begin narrating the incident into the AED's audio recorder. You continue this narration throughout the entire incident.

After several seconds of analysis, the AED issues a "SHOCK" message. Realizing that the patient is in a shockable state of cardiac arrest, you state, "Prepare for defibrillation. Everybody clear the patient!" All team members promptly comply. With everyone clear, you press the SHOCK button. The patient appears to jump slightly as the first shock is delivered. One of your team members starts to check for a pulse; however, you order him not to, as this will only delay further heart analysis and defibrillation if needed. Again, you clear all rescuers from the patient and press the ANALYZE button.

Once again, the AED gives a "SHOCK" message. You clear everyone from the patient and deliver a second defibrillating shock. Immediately, you press the ANALYZE button for reanalysis of the patient's heart. This time, a "NO SHOCK" message is returned.

Realizing that the patient may have regained a pulse or may be in a non-shockable state of cardiac arrest, you order a team member to check for a carotid pulse. He states excitedly that he can feel a pulse! He further states that the patient is breathing adequately but still appears unresponsive.

As there is no evidence of traumatic neck injury, the patient is placed in the recovery position. The third team member performs an assessment every thirty seconds. The patient maintains a pulse and breathing and begins to regain consciousness. You make note of these changes on the AED's built-in audio recorder.

(continued)

> Within minutes, the advanced care ambulance arrives. As the paramedics assume care, you inform them that the patient was found in cardiac arrest and after two defibrillating shocks regained a pulse and began breathing.
>
> The paramedics start an IV and deliver medical oxygen via a face mask. They administer some emergency drugs to the patient and load him for transport to a local hospital. Three weeks later he is released.

For example: "We have a sixty-two-year-old male patient who was found unresponsive, breathless, and without a pulse. We immediately applied the AED and received a "SHOCK" message. The AED delivered two shocks, after which a "NO SHOCK" message was given. A pulse was not present so we performed CPR and reanalyzed the patient's heart at one-minute intervals. He has remained in a nonshockable state ever since. At this time, we are continuing CPR."

SUMMARY

Once early access has occurred, the cardiac arrest patient's best hope for survival lies in the smooth and organized delivery of care. If the patient assessment reveals cardiac arrest, rapid application and operation of the AED must follow. If shockable cardiac arrest is identified, provide immediate defibrillating shocks with the AED.

As stressed throughout this book, defibrillation can never occur too early! The longer shockable cardiac arrest persists, the less likely that defibrillating shocks will be able to convert it into a heartbeat capable of pumping blood. *Every second counts when applying and using the AED!*

Keep in mind that when working with other rescuers, leadership and teamwork are the basis of quality care. Typically, operation of the AED is given to the person with the greatest knowledge and competence regarding cardiac arrest resuscitation and the AED. Accordingly, overall scene direction is best placed with the operator of the AED. As the AED operator, you must be effective at delegating and supervising all aspects of cardiac arrest resuscitation while simultaneously using the AED. Every rescuer must be dedicated to a team approach, as the patient's best chance for survival lies in cooperation.

FOOD FOR THOUGHT

To test your understanding, read and discuss the following questions.

1. *You assess an unresponsive female and find her to be breathing adequately with a strong pulse. There are no indications of a traumatic neck injury. What emergency care will you give this patient?*

   Remember that you can apply an AED only to a patient who is in cardiac arrest. Since the unresponsive female is breathing adequately and has a strong pulse, she is not in cardiac arrest. Therefore, do not apply the AED! Rather, notify advanced care if you haven't already done so, and place the patient in the recovery position. Administer medical oxygen with a face mask, if available, and wait with the patient until advanced care personnel arrive.

2. *The AED has informed you that the patient you are caring for is in shockable cardiac arrest. Why is it important to clear everyone from the patient prior to defibrillating?*

   Defibrillation involves the delivery of an electrical current to the heart of a person in cardiac arrest. The patient's body can conduct that current to anyone who is in physical contact with him or her. Although an electrical shock is beneficial for a heart in cardiac arrest, it can be dangerous to a heart that is pumping blood. If accidentally shocked, a rescuer may suffer injury or even go into cardiac arrest! Consequently, it is important to clear everybody from the patient before defibrillating.

3. *You have just delivered the third and final shock of a first set of stacked shocks. What should your next action be?*

   After delivering the third and final stacked shock, you must immediately check for a carotid pulse. If you find a pulse, you should check to see if the patient is breathing. If the patient is breathing adequately and you do not suspect a neck injury, place the patient in the recovery position and administer medical oxygen with a face mask, if available. If you suspect a traumatic neck injury, hold the patient's head, neck, and back in a straight position and wait for advanced care to arrive.

   If the patient has regained a pulse but is not breathing adequately, begin rescue breathing as described in Appendix A. The use of a pocket mask or face shield is recommended.

   If the patient has not regained a pulse, perform one minute of CPR. After one minute of CPR, reanalyze the patient's heart with the AED.

Defibrillate if a "SHOCK" message is received. If a "NO SHOCK" message is returned, check for a carotid pulse. If you find a pulse, continue as described above. If a pulse has not returned, perform one minute of CPR and reanalyze the patient's heart with the AED.

4. *After delivering two stacked shocks, the AED issues a "NO SHOCK" message. You immediately check for a carotid pulse and discover that one has returned. What should you do at this point? What would you do if you could not find a pulse following the "NO SHOCK" message?*

After receiving a "NO SHOCK" message and finding a pulse, immediately check for breathing. An adequately breathing patient whom you do not suspect has suffered a neck injury should be placed in the recovery position with medical oxygen administered through a face mask, if available. If the patient is not adequately breathing, start rescue breaths as described in Appendix A. If you suspect a neck injury, hold the patient's head, neck, and back in a straight line and wait until advanced care arrives. Deliver rescue breaths if needed.

If after receiving a "NO SHOCK" message you cannot locate a carotid pulse, perform one minute of CPR. After one minute of CPR, reanalyze the patient's heart with the AED. Administer a shock if a "SHOCK" message is received. If a "NO SHOCK" message is returned, check for a carotid pulse. If you find a pulse, continue as described previously. If a pulse has not returned, perform one minute of CPR and reanalyze the patient's heart with the AED.

REFERENCES

American Heart Association. (1998). *Heartsaver AED for the lay rescuer and first responder.* Dallas: Author.

Bergeron, J. D., & Bizjak, G. (1999). *First responder* (5th ed.). Upper Saddle River, NJ: Prentice Hall.

Hafen, B. Q., Karren, K. J., & Mistovich, J. J. (1996). *Prehospital emergency care* (5th ed.). Upper Saddle River, NJ: Prentice Hall.

United States Department of Transportation. (1994). *EMT basic national standard curricula.* Washington, DC: Government Printing Office.

7

Special Resuscitative Situations

LEARNING OBJECTIVES

At the end of this chapter, you will be able to

- Identify the corrective actions to take if you encounter the hazards of water and metal
- Describe the guidelines for determining whether a child in cardiac arrest should receive treatment with an AED
- Describe the special considerations for treating a cardiac arrest patient with a pacemaker or an automatic implantable cardiac defibrillator
- Describe the special care given to a hypothermic patient in cardiac arrest
- Describe the measures taken when advanced care is not available
- Identify the special considerations for using an AED while transporting a cardiac patient
- Describe the measures taken when a cardiac arrest patient has a medication patch on his or her chest

---

KEY TERMS

Cardiac pacemaker—A mechanical device that electrically stimulates the heart to beat and pump blood.

Automated implantable cardiac defibrillator (AICD)—A small defibrillator that is internally attached to the wall of the heart.

Hypothermia—A state in which the internal body temperature is below normal.

Medication patch—A small patch containing medication, which is absorbed through the skin. Medication patches are frequently placed on the chest.

As a provider of emergency cardiac care, you may encounter unusual circumstances that change the way you will deliver care with an AED. This chapter presents some of these situations and describes the correct alternate care to use.

HANDLING WATER AND METAL HAZARDS

If the cardiac arrest patient is located in water or on a metal surface, administering a defibrillating shock would be dangerous to both the patient and the rescuer. Water and metal conduct electricity. If a patient in water or on metal is shocked, the electrical current can be transferred to anyone in contact with that water or metal.

As stressed throughout this book, although a defibrillating shock can be beneficial to a heart in cardiac arrest, it can be extremely dangerous to a heart *not* in cardiac arrest. *An accidental shock may cause injury to the rescuer!* Therefore, it is important that the AED operator actively look for water and metal hazards.

If a person in cardiac arrest is located in water, *rapidly* move him or her to a dry location. If the patient is wet, quickly dry his or her chest before applying the adhesive electrodes. Drying the chest will help the electrodes adhere and will prevent the conduction of electricity over the surface of the chest between the two electrodes. If the cardiac arrest patient is positioned on a metal surface, quickly remove him or her to a safer area before applying the AED.

TREATING INFANTS AND CHILDREN

Most AEDs are programmed to deliver shocks to an adult patient. The larger heart of an adult requires more electricity per shock than does the smaller heart of an infant or small child. An AED can deliver an excessive amount of electricity to a young child or infant, possibly damaging the heart. Therefore, the American Heart Association (1998) recommends that an AED should be used only on children who are eight years of age or older.

If you are presented with an infant or child that is younger than eight years, initiate CPR and notify advanced care as quickly as possible. (*Note:* Some sources, such as the United States Department of Transportation, set the age limit at twelve years or a weight greater than 90 pounds, or 40 kilograms [United States Department of Transportation, 1994]. Follow local guidelines.)

TREATING PATIENTS WITH CARDIAC PACEMAKERS AND AUTOMATIC IMPLANTABLE CARDIAC DEFIBRILLATORS

Patients with chronic heart problems may have electrical devices implanted directly into the heart. The most common of these devices are the **cardiac pacemaker** and the **automatic implantable cardiac defibrillator (AICD)**. The presence of either device slightly alters the way care is provided with an AED.

Cardiac Pacemakers

Cardiac pacemakers provide a regular heartbeat to individuals whose hearts beat too slowly or irregularly. The pacemaker is implanted directly into the heart and has a separate power source, usually located underneath the skin below the left collarbone. The power source is evidenced by a bulge in the skin in this location.

Placing an AED's electrodes over the top of a pacemaker's power source can result in an ineffective defibrillation. To deliver an effective defibrillation, ensure that the adhesive electrodes are not over the top of the power source but at least one inch away from it (American Heart Association, 1998).

Automated Implantable Cardiac Defibrillators

An AICD is a defibrillator that is implanted directly into the heart of a patient at high risk for cardiac arrest. Similar to the AED, an AICD continually monitors the heart and will quickly defibrillate it if it goes into a shockable state of cardiac arrest. When the AICD defibrillates, contraction of the chest muscles occurs.

If confronted with a conscious and breathing patient with an AICD that is actively defibrillating, *do not* apply the AED! Observe the chest wall for contractions caused by internal defibrillation, and evaluate the patient for a sudden loss of consciousness. The AICD delivers a small amount of electricity that does not pose a threat to you if you touch the patient.

If the patient becomes unresponsive, assess the patient for cardiac arrest. If the patient is unresponsive, breathless, and without a pulse, look for chest wall contraction associated with internal defibrillation. If no contractions are observable, the AICD is not actively defibrillating. Apply and use your AED in customary fashion.

If contractions are evident, wait for the contractions associated with defibrillation to stop. Once the contractions stop, assess the patient for cardiac arrest. If the patient is still in cardiac arrest, apply and use the AED. If the patient is not in cardiac arrest, do not apply the AED but render supportive care. The power source for the AICD is generally located on the chest of the left side of the abdomen. As with the pacemaker, do not place the AED electrodes over the top of the AICD's power source but one inch away from it (American Heart Association, 1998).

TREATING PATIENTS WITH HYPOTHERMIA

Hypothermia occurs when a person's body temperature drops well below normal (*hypo* means "below"; *thermia* refers to "temperature"). Prolonged exposure to cold is a common cause of hypothermia. A hypothermic patient is cold to the touch.

A cold heart in shockable cardiac arrest is difficult to convert with a defibrillating shock. Many times, careful rewarming in a medical facility must occur, as the warmer heart is more receptive to defibrillation.

The American Heart Association recommends that when treating a hypothermic patient in cardiac arrest, you should deliver up to three stacked shocks if the patient is in a shockable state. If after the third shock the patient remains in shockable cardiac arrest, withhold further shocks (American Heart Association, 1997). Continue CPR while arranging for transport to a medical facility where rewarming can take place. The coldness of the body preserves the cells and organs for longer periods. Follow local guidelines concerning hypothermia and use of the AED.

TREATING PATIENTS WHEN ADVANCED CARE IS NOT AVAILABLE

Any patient that has been successfully defibrillated or remains in nonshockable cardiac arrest requires advanced care. However, there may be times when advanced care is delayed or not available.

If the AED team has the ability to transport the patient (in an ambulance or other authorized vehicle), they should do so once the patient has regained a pulse or if the patient remains in cardiac arrest despite resuscitative efforts. If you do not have transport capabilities, remain with the patient until a means of transport arrives. In both cases, continue appropriate care throughout. Follow local guidelines concerning the unavailability of advanced care.

TREATING PATIENTS DURING TRANSPORT

Some AED rescue teams have the capability to transport a cardiac patient. If use of the AED is required during transport, special measures must be taken.

If you are transporting a conscious patient who suddenly becomes unresponsive, stop the vehicle and assess the patient by evaluating his or her airway, breathing, and circulation. If the patient is in cardiac arrest, initiate CPR (if more than one rescuer is present) and apply the AED. Use the AED as described in Chapter Six. Resume transport if one of the following three criteria are met:

- The patient regains a pulse
- The patient remains in a shockable state of cardiac arrest after a preestablished number of shocks have been delivered (follow local guidelines)
- Three consecutive "NO SHOCK" messages are received

Continue care as described in Chapter Six. As a general rule, *stop the vehicle every time the AED is placed in analysis mode or delivers a defibrillating shock!* (Some authorities recommend turning the vehicle's engine off during analysis and defibrillation with an AED. Refer to manufacturer recommendations concerning this matter.) Notify advanced care at the earliest possible moment.

If transporting an unresponsive patient who is breathing and has a pulse, continually assess the patient, using the ABCs of assessment, for signs of cardiac arrest. If the patient goes into cardiac arrest, use the AED as previously described. Resume transport if one of the above three criteria is satisfied.

TREATING PATIENTS WITH TRAUMATIC CARDIAC ARREST

Serious injuries (such as those sustained in an automobile accident, a shooting, a stabbing, or a fall from a high place) can cause traumatic cardiac arrest. In traumatic cardiac arrest, the primary problem is the loss of blood or damage to the body, not cardiac compromise as is the case in general cardiac arrest. With traumatic cardiac arrest, the heart is most frequently in a nonshockable state. Even if the heart is in a shockable state, successful defibrillation often proves difficult.

Some authorities recommend that traumatic cardiac arrest not be treated with an AED. A patient in traumatic cardiac arrest requires rapid transport to a hospital for surgical repair and blood administration, and taking time to apply and use an AED only serves to delay that transport (if it is available) and treatment. Other authorities do not differentiate general cardiac arrest from traumatic cardiac arrest and recommend that an AED be used to treat both types. *Follow local guidelines concerning this matter.*

Do not confuse traumatic neck injury with traumatic cardiac arrest. Traumatic neck injuries are suffered after the onset of cardiac arrest when the patient loses consciousness and falls to the ground, striking the head or neck. These injuries follow the onset of cardiac arrest, as opposed to traumatic cardiac arrest, where the injury causes the cardiac arrest.

Treating Patients with a Medication Patch

If the patient has a **medication patch** on his or her chest, remove it before defibrillating. Medication patches may have a metal or plastic backing that can interfere with the delivery of a defibrillating shock. Additionally, the patch may melt and cause burns to the patient's skin (American Heart Association, 1998).

Summary

Special situations may require you to modify the standard treatment given with an AED. As a rescuer, you must be familiar with these situations and prepared to take the necessary corrective actions. By your doing so, the best possible cardiac care will be delivered, giving the patient the greatest possible chance for recovery.

Food for Thought

To test your understanding, read and discuss the following questions.

1. *You arrive on the scene of a cardiac arrest in a parking lot following a heavy rainstorm. You see several rescuers standing in a large puddle about to defibrillate the patient, who lies in the same puddle. What should you immediately do, and why?*

   Water poses a hazard to both the patient and the rescuer when an AED is being used. If a patient is in contact with water, the electrical current from the AED can be transferred to anyone else in contact with that water. Although a defibrillating shock is beneficial for a heart in a shockable form of cardiac arrest, it can cause injury to a heart that is not in cardiac arrest. In this scenario, you would not enter the water but would immediately shout a warning to warn the rescuers of the danger.

2. *At an AED community awareness meeting, a citizen asks you why your AED cannot be used to defibrillate a small child who is less than eight years of age. What would you tell him?*

   Most AEDs are designed to administer shocks to an adult in cardiac arrest. Adults' hearts are larger and require more electrical energy to restart than do the hearts of children. Delivering an excessive amount of electricity to a child's heart can damage the heart and actually worsen the chance of recovery. Therefore, the American Heart Association recommends that AEDs not be used on children who are younger than eight years of age. (The U.S.

Department of Transportation [1994] sets the age limit at twelve years and the weight threshold at 90 pounds.) Follow local guidelines concerning this matter.

3. *As a member of a ski patrol, you have been summoned to the side of a hypothermic man in cardiac arrest. After applying an AED and analyzing the man's heart, you find him in shockable cardiac arrest. Assuming that the patient remains in shockable cardiac arrest, how will you treat this patient?*

A cold heart in shockable cardiac arrest can be difficult to treat with defibrillation. Often, rewarming in a medical facility must first take place before the heart will respond to defibrillation with an AED. When treating a hypothermic patient in shockable cardiac arrest, deliver the initial set of up to three stacked shocks. If the patient remains in a shockable state of cardiac arrest following these three shocks, withhold further shocks and perform CPR while awaiting advanced care or making arrangements for transport to a medical facility where rewarming can take place. If the patient converts to nonshockable cardiac arrest, continue CPR and wait for advanced care or transport to a medical facility.

4. *You have come to the assistance of an elderly male in cardiac arrest. When cutting away his shirt, you notice a medication patch on the left side of his chest. Why must you remove the medication patch before defibrillating with the AED?*

The medication patch on the patient's chest can interfere with the delivery of an effective shock or cause the patient injury if defibrillation is required. Some medication patches have a metal or plastic backing. The electricity from a defibrillating shock can melt the backing, causing burns to the patient's chest. Therefore, a medication patch should be removed from the chest of any cardiac arrest patient.

REFERENCES

American Heart Association. (1997). *Basic life support for healthcare providers.* Dallas: Author.

American Heart Association. (1998). *Heartsaver AED for the lay rescuer and first responder.* Dallas: Author.

United States Department of Transportation. (1994). *EMT basic national standard curricula.* Washington, DC: Government Printing Office.

8

Application Exercises

In cases of cardiac arrest, time is of the essence, as the brain, heart, and other organs begin to die once circulation of oxygenated blood ceases. Therefore, rapid identification of cardiac arrest and swift treatment with an AED are critical in emergency cardiac care. The best emergency care is proficient emergency care. Proficiency saves time. To become proficient, you must practice.

SCENARIO-BASED APPLICATION EXERCISES

The following pages provide scenario-based exercises to help you practice administering emergency care with an AED. The scenarios provide a brief description of the cardiac emergency and outcome. In between, you are asked to supply the emergency care needed to achieve this outcome. To complete these exercises, verbally describe or physically act out, in the correct order, the correct procedures for patient assessment, CPR, and AED operation.

In some scenarios the rescuer must act alone, whereas others involve a team approach. In team-oriented scenarios, you must act as team leader and delegate patient care tasks while simultaneously operating the AED. In all scenarios, an SAED is used, as it is the more common of the two types of AEDs.

Compare the treatment you provide with the corresponding emergency care summaries later in this chapter. These summaries identify each step in the correct order. Use them as a guide and feedback on your performance.

Scenario 1: Person Down in the Parking Lot

You are employed as an AED technician at an emergency care center. The other employees have gone for lunch, leaving you by yourself. Suddenly a woman bangs on the door, shouting that a man is lying face down in the parking lot. You grab your AED and rush to the patient's side. As you approach the patient, you do not observe any signs indicating a neck injury. You perform the ABCs of patient assessment and find that the man is unresponsive but is breathing adequately and has a pulse.

- Describe or physically enact the individual steps of emergency care up to a determination that the patient is not in cardiac arrest.
- Describe or physically enact the individual steps of emergency care that follow your determination that the patient is not in cardiac arrest. Assume that the patient remains breathing adequately and with a pulse.
- Compare your actions with the emergency care summary later in this chapter.

Scenario 2: Gentleman Collapsed in the Lobby

You are certified as an emergency AED health care provider and work in the county government building. While walking to the copy machine, you discover an elderly gentleman on his back in the lobby. You shout for help and retrieve a nearby AED. While returning to the patient, you instruct a security guard to call 911 and request an EMS/advanced care ambulance. Two other coworkers, also certified in AED operation, have heard you call and come to assist you.

As you and your coworkers approach the patient, you do not observe any signs indicating a neck injury. At the patient's side, the first rescuer performs the ABCs of patient assessment as you prepare the AED. After assessing the patient, the first rescuer states that the patient is in cardiac arrest. In addition, he informs you that the patient has a power source for a pacemaker below his left collarbone. Following application and activation of the AED, you receive a "NO SHOCK" message. The carotid pulse remains absent.

- Describe or physically enact the individual steps of emergency care up to a determination that the patient is in nonshockable cardiac arrest.
- Describe or physically enact the individual steps of emergency care after determining that the patient is in nonshockable cardiac arrest. Assume that the patient remains in nonshockable cardiac arrest.
- Compare your actions with the emergency care summary later in the chapter.

Scenario 3: Early Defibrillation in the Hospital

As a registered nurse working in a small hospital, you have been certified in the use of an AED. Late one evening you hear a cry for help down the hall. Anticipating a cardiac problem, you and another nurse grab an AED and instruct a ward clerk to notify the emergency department to send advanced care personnel and equipment. Quickly you proceed down the hallway and find a sixty-year-old male patient lying face down on the floor. Blood appears to be coming from a laceration above his right eye. An orderly who witnessed the event states that the laceration occurred when the man collapsed and struck his head on a chair.

Your coworker performs the ABCs of patient assessment and declares him to be in cardiac arrest. Quickly you ready and apply the AED. After the delivery of two defibrillatory shocks, a "NO SHOCK" message is received. The patient remains in cardiac arrest.

- Describe or physically enact the individual steps of emergency care up to and including the delivery of two defibrillating shocks.
- Describe or physically enact the individual steps of emergency care that will follow the delivery of two defibrillating shocks and the onset of nonshockable cardiac arrest. Assume that the patient remains in nonshockable cardiac arrest.
- Compare your actions with the emergency care summary later in the chapter.

Scenario 4: Cardiac Arrest in a High-Rise

Your employers are committed to providing a safer workplace and have instituted an emergency AED program, for which you have been designated the primary operator. While at work, you witness the collapse of a building custodian. Quickly you retrieve an AED and instruct a coworker to call 911 and request an ambulance with paramedics capable of delivering advanced care.

You reach the custodian's side and observe him face up on the floor. There are no signs indicating a neck injury. Without any help, you quickly perform the ABCs of patient assessment. The man is in cardiac arrest. Knowing that seconds count, you quickly prepare and apply the AED. After receiving a "SHOCK" message, you deliver one shock. A "NO SHOCK" message follows, and you discover that although still unresponsive, the custodian has regained a pulse and is breathing adequately.

- Describe or physically enact the individual steps of emergency care up to a return of a patient's pulse and adequate breathing.
- Describe or physically enact each step of emergency care that must follow the successful defibrillation. Assume that the custodian remains breathing and with a pulse.
- Compare your actions with the emergency care summary later in the chapter.

Scenario 5: First Responder Defibrillation

As an AED first responder, you and a partner have been placed on standby at a local festival to which thousands of patrons have flocked. Over the radio, you are instructed to proceed to the vending area, where a person has collapsed. The dispatcher states that paramedics capable of providing advanced care are being dispatched.

On location, you observe an elderly female lying on her back in the grass. Bystanders state that the patient was sitting down when she suddenly lost consciousness. A friend prevented her from falling and placed her on the grass. Consequently, there is no possibility of a neck injury.

Your partner assesses the patient and confirms that she is in cardiac arrest. You apply the AED and deliver three shocks. After the third shock, you find that the patient is breathing adequately and with a pulse but is still unresponsive.

- Describe or physically enact the individual steps of emergency care up to a return of a spontaneous pulse and adequate breathing.
- Describe or physically enact the steps of emergency care that must follow the successful defibrillation. Assume that the patient remains with a pulse and adequate breathing.
- Compare your actions with the emergency care summary later in the chapter.

Scenario 6: Cardiac Arrest in a Casino

A large casino employs you as an AED emergency caregiver. While making rounds, you are alerted to a woman who appears sick. You obtain an AED, and after a two-minute walk you discover a woman on her back on the floor with a large laceration on the forehead, sustained when she fell. You immediately assess the patient and instruct a security guard to call for advanced care assistance. Assessment reveals the patient to be in cardiac arrest.

After applying the AED and delivering a total of four defibrillating shocks, the patient regains a spontaneous pulse and adequate breathing. Unfortunately, you do not have any assistance and must work alone.

- Describe or physically enact the individual steps of emergency care up to a return of a spontaneous pulse and breathing.
- Describe or physically enact the steps of emergency care that must follow the successful defibrillation. Assume that the patient remains with a pulse and adequate breathing.
- Compare your actions with the emergency care summary later in the chapter. *Hint: defibrillatory shocks with an AED are delivered in individual sets of up to three stacked shocks.*

Scenario 7: Cardiac Arrest at a Sporting Event

As a police officer certified to use an AED, you are working at a large sporting event involving thousands of spectators. Everything is calm until you are told of an unresponsive person in a car in the parking lot. You radio for advanced care assistance and grab an AED. Since the parking lot is only a short distance from your base, you and a partner run to the location and find a male slumped over the wheel of a parked vehicle. As you approach the patient, you see no signs indicating a neck injury. Your partner quickly performs the ABCs of patient assessment. He informs you that the man is in cardiac arrest. You quickly prepare and apply the AED.

Although you are a seasoned AED operator, this resuscitation proves to be the most complicated one you've ever attempted. After four defibrillating shocks, a "NO SHOCK" message is received. The pulse remains absent. During reanalysis, the AED advises that the patient is once again in a shockable state. After the delivery of a fifth shock, the patient regains a pulse and adequate breathing and begins to regain consciousness.

- Describe or physically enact the individual steps of emergency care up to a return of a spontaneous pulse and breathing.
- Describe or physically enact the steps of emergency care that must follow the successful defibrillation. Assume that the patient remains with a pulse and breathing.
- Compare your actions with the emergency care summary later in the chapter.

EMERGENCY CARE SUMMARIES

The following pages contain emergency care summaries for the seven scenario-based exercises just presented. Each summary lists the individual steps of emergency care in the order in which they should be performed. Use the emergency care summary for guidance or feedback on your performance.

Scenario 1

Scenario 1 presents an unresponsive patient who is not in cardiac arrest. *Do not apply the AED to the patient!* Remember that you are by yourself, with no one to provide assistance. To determine that the patient is not in cardiac arrest, take the following steps:

1. *Obtain the AED.* Quickly obtain the AED and instruct the woman to activate the EMS/advanced care system.

2. *Size up the scene.* Ensure that the scene is safe, and take BSI measures (gloves and protective face and eyewear). Quickly scan the patient for signs indicating a possible neck injury as you approach. In this scenario you find no such signs.

3. *Assess the patient.* Determine unresponsiveness by shaking the patient and shouting, "Can you hear me? Are you okay?" The patient is unresponsive. Carefully roll the patient onto his back and continue with the assessment. In this order, perform the steps of patient assessment:
   - Check the patient's airway. Open the airway by performing the head tilt–chin lift maneuver.
   - Check the patient's breathing. Look, listen, and feel for breathing. The patient is breathing adequately.
   - Check the patient's circulation. Check for a carotid pulse. A carotid pulse is felt.

Although unresponsive, the patient is breathing adequately and has a pulse. Therefore, the patient is not in cardiac arrest and the AED must not be applied. Rather, focus emergency care on maintaining an open airway and continual reassessment until advanced care personnel arrive. Perform the following steps of emergency care:

4. Place the patient in the recovery position.
5. *Reassess the patient.* Continually reassess the patient by evaluating responsiveness and the ABCs. If it is available, administer medical oxygen with a face mask. Wait with the patient until advanced care personnel arrive.

Scenario 2

In this scenario, the patient is in a nonshockable state of cardiac arrest and will not benefit from a defibrillating shock. In addition, the patient has a pacemaker, with the power source located below the left collarbone. The steps needed to determine nonshockable cardiac arrest are as follows:

1. *Obtain the AED.* Quickly obtain the AED and instruct the security guard to activate the EMS/advanced care system.
2. *Size up the scene.* Ensure that the scene is safe, and take BSI measures (gloves and protective face and eyewear). Quickly scan the patient for signs indicating a possible neck injury as you approach. In this scenario, you find no such signs.
3. *Assess the patient and prepare the AED.* Instruct your coworker to determine patient unresponsiveness by shaking the patient and shouting "Can

you hear me? Are you okay?" The patient is unresponsive. As team leader, you start preparing the AED for application. Have a coworker complete the assessment by performing the following steps, in the order listed:

- Check the patient's airway. Open the airway by performing the head tilt–chin lift maneuver.
- Check the patient's breathing. Look, listen, and feel for breathing. The patient is breathless. Deliver two rescue breaths.
- Check the patient's circulation. Check for a carotid pulse. No pulse is felt.

The patient is in cardiac arrest; therefore, fast application of the AED is critical. As you have two coworkers assisting you, delegate all tasks not directly associated with the AED and its operation.

4. *Initiate CPR.* Instruct your coworkers to initiate CPR. *As the AED operator, do not stop preparation of the AED to assist with CPR!* This will delay the application and use of the AED.
5. *Apply the AED.* Turn on the AED and apply the electrodes to the patient's chest. Make sure that the electrodes are at least one inch away from the power source of the pacemaker.
6. *Analyze the patient's heart.* Ensure that all rescuers are clear of the patient, and press the ANALYZE button to analyze the patient's heart. A "NO SHOCK" message is received.
7. *Check the patient's pulse.* Check for a carotid pulse. No pulse is felt. State "No pulse present. The patient is in nonshockable cardiac arrest!"
8. *Again perform CPR.* Instruct your coworkers to perform CPR for one minute.
9. *Reanalyze the heart.* Stop CPR after one minute and clear both coworkers from the patient. Do not check for a pulse, but press the ANALYZE button to reanalyze the patient's heart. A "NO SHOCK" message is received.

Assuming that the patient remains in nonshockable cardiac arrest, emergency care should continue as follows:

10. *Check the patient's pulse.* Check for a carotid pulse. No pulse is felt. State "No pulse present. The patient is still in nonshockable cardiac arrest!"
11. *Again perform CPR.* Instruct the team members to perform CPR for one minute.
12. *Reanalyze the patient's heart and check the pulse.* Stop CPR after one minute and clear all rescuers from the patient. Reanalyze the patient's heart. A "NO SHOCK" message is received. Check for a carotid pulse. No pulse is felt.

After three consecutive "NO SHOCK" messages, reanalysis of the heart can be performed at one- to two-minute intervals, with CPR occurring between. At this point, the return of shockable cardiac arrest is unlikely. Continue CPR until advanced care personnel arrive.

Scenario 3

In this scenario, the cardiac arrest patient initially presents with a shockable form of cardiac arrest. After two shocks, however, a "NO SHOCK" message is returned, as the patient has lapsed into a nonshockable state of cardiac arrest. Here are the steps for this scenario, in order:

1. *Obtain the AED.* Quickly obtain the AED and move toward the patient's location. Instruct your coworker to contact the Emergency Department for advanced care assistance.
2. *Size up the scene.* Ensure a safe scene and take BSI measures (gloves and protective face and eyewear). Quickly scan the patient for signs indicating a possible neck injury as you approach. In this scenario, the patient struck his head when he collapsed, as evidenced by the laceration above his right eye. Therefore, the possibility of a neck injury exists. Take all neck injury precautions.
3. *Assess the patient and prepare the AED.* As team leader, you instruct your coworker to stabilize the head and neck and determine unresponsiveness by shouting "Can you hear me? Are you okay?" The patient is unresponsive. Carefully roll the patient onto his back by moving the head, neck, and back as one unit. As leader, you prepare the AED for application and use. Have your coworker complete the patient assessment by performing the following steps as listed.
   • Check the patient's airway. Open the airway by performing the jaw-thrust maneuver. Do not use the head tilt–chin lift maneuver, because of possible neck injury.
   • Check the patient's breathing. Look, listen, and feel for breathing. The patient is breathless. Deliver two rescue breaths.
   • Check the patient's circulation. Check for a carotid pulse. No pulse is felt.

The patient is in cardiac arrest; therefore, fast application of the AED is critical. Since you have assistance, delegate all tasks not directly associated with the AED and its operation:

4. *Initiate CPR.* Instruct your coworker to initiate CPR. *As AED operator, do not stop preparation of the AED to assist with CPR!* This will delay the application and use of the AED.

5. *Apply the AED.* Turn on the AED and apply the electrodes to the patient's chest.
6. *Analyze the patient's heart.* Ensure that your coworker is clear of the patient, and press the ANALYZE button to analyze the patient's heart. A "SHOCK" message is received.
7. *Deliver a shock.* Ensure that your coworker is clear of the patient, and press the SHOCK button to deliver the first shock.
8. *Reanalyze the patient's heart.* Do not check for a pulse, but reanalyze the patient's heart. A "SHOCK" message is received.
9. *Deliver another shock.* Ensure that your coworker is clear of the patient, and press the SHOCK button to deliver a second shock.
10. *Reanalyze the heart.* Do not check for a pulse, but immediately reanalyze the patient's heart. A "NO SHOCK" message is received.
11. *Check the patient's pulse.* Check for a carotid pulse. No pulse is felt. State "No pulse is present. The patient is in nonshockable cardiac arrest!"

Assuming that the patient remains in nonshockable cardiac arrest, the following emergency care should be performed:

12. *Perform CPR.* Instruct your coworker to perform CPR for one minute.
13. *Reanalyze the heart.* Stop CPR after one minute and clear your coworker from the patient. Do not check for a pulse, but immediately reanalyze the patient's heart. A "NO SHOCK" message is received.
14. *Check the patient's pulse.* Check for a carotid pulse. No pulse is found. State *"No pulse is present. The patient is still in nonshockable cardiac arrest!"*
15. *Perform CPR.* Instruct your coworker to perform CPR for one minute.
16. *Reanalyze the heart.* Stop CPR after one minute and clear your coworker from the patient. Reanalyze the patient's heart. A "NO SHOCK" message is received. Check for a carotid pulse. No pulse is found as the patient remains in nonshockable cardiac arrest. Continue CPR for one minute and then reanalyze the heart again.

After three consecutive "NO SHOCK" messages, reanalysis of the heart can be performed at one- to two-minute intervals, with CPR occurring between. At this point, the return of shockable cardiac arrest is unlikely. Continue management until advanced care personnel arrive.

Scenario 4

In this scenario, the patient has been successfully defibrillated and, even though unresponsive, has a strong pulse and adequate breathing. *Remember that you are alone and without help.* Perform these steps, in this order:

1. *Obtain the AED.* Quickly obtain the AED and move toward the patient's location. Instruct a coworker to call 911 and request EMS/advanced care assistance.
2. *Size up the scene.* Ensure a safe scene and take BSI measures (gloves and protective face and eyewear). Quickly scan the patient for signs indicating a possible neck injury as you approach. In this scenario, you find no such signs.
3. *Assess the patient.* Determine unresponsiveness by shaking the patient and shouting, "Can you hear me? Are you okay?" The patient is unresponsive. Perform the following steps of patient assessment, in order:
   • Check the patient's airway. Open the airway by performing the head tilt–chin lift maneuver.
   • Check the patient's breathing. Look, listen, and feel for breathing. The patient is breathless. Deliver two rescue breaths.
   • Check the patient's circulation. Check for a carotid pulse. No pulse is felt.

The patient is in cardiac arrest; therefore, fast application of the AED is critical. *Since you are alone, do not perform CPR!* The priority remains application of the AED. Quickly do the following:

4. *Prepare and apply the AED.* Turn on the AED and apply the electrodes to the patient's chest.
5. *Analyze the patient's heart.* Ensure that you are clear of the patient, and press the ANALYZE button to analyze the patient's heart. A "SHOCK" message is received.
6. *Deliver a shock.* Ensure that you are clear of the patient, and press the SHOCK button to deliver the first shock.
7. *Reanalyze the patient's heart.* Do not check for a pulse, but immediately reanalyze the patient's heart. A "NO SHOCK" message is received.
8. *Check the patient's pulse.* Check for a carotid pulse. A carotid pulse is felt. State, *"The patient has regained a pulse!"*

Since the patient has regained a pulse, continue care as follows:

9. *Check the patient's breathing.* Assess for breathing. In addition to having a pulse, the patient is breathing adequately. (If the patient were not breathing or were breathing inadequately, you would administer rescue breaths at a rate of twelve per minute.)
10. *Place the patient in the recovery position.* Place the patient in the recovery position, as described previously.
11. *Reassess the patient.* Continually reevaluate the patient for any change in status by assessing responsiveness, airway, breathing, and circulation every

thirty seconds. Remember that the patient may fall back into cardiac arrest. Because the patient was just resuscitated from cardiac arrest, leave the AED in place. *Do not use the AED to reanalyze the patient's heart unless your assessment reveals that he has gone back into cardiac arrest!* If available, administer oxygen via a face mask. Wait with the patient until advanced care arrives.

If the patient relapses into cardiac arrest, use the AED as previously described.

Scenario 5

In this scenario, the patient has been successfully defibrillated from cardiac arrest and, even though unresponsive, is breathing adequately and has a pulse. Prior to the successful defibrillation, the following emergency care must be given:

1. *Obtain the AED.* Quickly obtain the AED and move toward the patient's location. The dispatcher has already requested EMS/advanced care assistance.
2. *Size up the scene.* Ensure a *safe* scene and take BSI measures (gloves and protective face and eyewear). Quickly scan the patient for signs of possible neck injury. In this scenario, you find no such signs.
3. *Assess the patient and prepare the AED.* Instruct a team member to determine unresponsiveness by shaking the patient and shouting "Can you hear me? Are you okay?" The patient is unresponsive. As team leader, you start preparing the AED for application. Have your partner continue by performing the ABCs of patient assessment:
    *   Check the patient's airway. Open the airway by performing the head tilt–chin lift maneuver.
    *   Check the patient's breathing. Look, listen, and feel for breathing. The patient is breathless. Deliver two rescue breaths.
    *   Check the patient's circulation. Check for a carotid pulse. No pulse is felt.

The patient is in cardiac arrest; therefore, fast application of the AED is critical. Since you have a partner to assist, delegate all tasks not directly associated with the AED and its operation:

4. *Initiate CPR.* Instruct your partner to initiate CPR. *As AED operator, do not stop preparation of the AED to assist with CPR!* This will delay the application of the AED.
5. *Apply the AED.* Turn on the AED and apply the electrodes to patient's chest.

6. *Analyze the patient's heart.* Clear your partner from the patient, and press the ANALYZE button to analyze the patient's heart. A "SHOCK" message is received.

7. *Deliver a shock.* Ensure that your partner is clear of the patient, and press the SHOCK button to deliver the first shock.

8. *Reanalyze the patient's heart.* Do not check for a pulse, but immediately reanalyze the patient's heart. A "SHOCK" message is received.

9. *Deliver another shock.* Ensure that your partner is clear of the patient, and press the SHOCK button to deliver the second shock.

10. *Reanalyze the patient's heart.* Do not check for a pulse, but immediately reanalyze the patient's heart. A "SHOCK" message is received.

11. *Deliver a third shock.* Ensure that your partner is clear of the patient, and press the SHOCK button to deliver the third and final shock of the first set of three stacked shocks.

12. *Check the patient's pulse.* Check for a carotid pulse. A carotid pulse is felt. State, *"The patient has regained a pulse!"*

Since the patient has regained a pulse, continue emergency care as follows:

13. *Check the patient's breathing.* Assess for breathing. In addition to having a pulse, the patient is breathing adequately. (If the patient were not breathing, you would administer rescue breaths at a rate of twelve per minute.)

14. *Place the patient in the recovery position.* Place the patient in the recovery position, as described previously.

15. *Reassess the patient.* Continually reevaluate the patient for any change in status by assessing responsiveness, airway, breathing, and circulation every thirty seconds. Remember that the patient may fall back into cardiac arrest. Because the patient was just resuscitated from cardiac arrest, leave the AED in place. *Do not use the AED to reanalyze the patient's heart unless your assessment reveals that the patient has gone back into cardiac arrest!* If available, administer oxygen via a face mask. Wait with the patient until advanced care arrives.

If the patient relapses into cardiac arrest, use the AED as previously described.

Scenario 6

In this scenario, the patient has been successfully resuscitated after four defibrillating shocks. *Remember that you are alone and without help.* Follow these steps, in order:

1. *Obtain the AED.* Obtain the AED and move toward the patient's location. Instruct the security guard to call for advanced care assistance.
2. *Size up the scene.* Ensure a safe scene and take BSI measures (gloves and protective face and eyewear). Quickly scan the patient for signs of a possible neck injury as you approach. In this scenario, a laceration on the patient's forehead indicates that she struck her head when she collapsed. Therefore, the possibility of a neck injury exists, and all neck injury precautions must be taken.
3. *Assess the patient.* Do not shake the patient, but hold her head still while shouting, "Can you hear me? Are you okay?" The patient is unresponsive. Complete the assessment as follows:
   - Check the patient's airway. Open the airway by performing the jaw-thrust maneuver. Do not perform the head tilt–chin lift maneuver, because of the possibility of neck injury.
   - Check the patient's breathing. Look, listen, and feel for breathing. The patient is breathless. Deliver two rescue breaths.
   - Check the patient's circulation. Check for a carotid pulse. No pulse is felt.

The patient is in cardiac arrest; therefore, fast application of the AED is critical. *Since you are alone, do not perform CPR!* The priority remains application of the AED:

4. *Prepare and apply the AED.* Turn on the AED and apply the electrodes to the patient's chest.
5. *Analyze the patient's heart.* Ensure that you are clear of the patient, and press the ANALYZE button to analyze the patient's heart. A "SHOCK" message is received.
6. *Deliver a shock.* Ensure that you are clear of the patient, and press the SHOCK button to deliver the first shock.
7. *Reanalyze the heart.* Do not check for a pulse, but immediately reanalyze the patient's heart. A "SHOCK" message is received.
8. *Deliver another shock.* Ensure that you are clear of the patient, and press the SHOCK button to deliver the second shock.
9. *Reanalyze the heart.* Do not check for a pulse, but immediately reanalyze the patient's heart. A "SHOCK" message is received.
10. *Deliver a third shock.* Ensure that you are clear of the patient, and press the SHOCK button to deliver the third and final shock.

A full set of three stacked shocks has been delivered. Before reanalyzing the heart, one minute of CPR is needed to perfuse the body's cells with oxygen-rich blood. Continue with the following care.

11. *Check the patient's pulse.* Check for a carotid pulse. No pulse is felt. State "No pulse is present. The patient is still in cardiac arrest!"
12. *Perform CPR.* Perform CPR for one minute.
13. *Reanalyze the heart.* Stop CPR after one minute. Do not check for a pulse, but immediately reanalyze the patient's heart. A "SHOCK" message is received.
14. *Deliver a fourth shock.* Ensure that you are clear of the patient, and press the SHOCK button to deliver a fourth shock.
15. *Reanalyze the patient's heart.* Do not check for a pulse, but immediately reanalyze the patient's heart. A "NO SHOCK" message is received.
16. *Check the patient's pulse.* Check for a carotid pulse. A carotid pulse is felt! State, "The patient has regained a pulse!"

As the patient has regained a pulse, emergency care should continue as follows:

17. *Check the patient's breathing.* Assess the patient for breathing. In addition to having a pulse, the patient is breathing adequately. (If the patient were not breathing, you would administer rescue breaths at a rate of twelve per minute.)
18. *Reassess the patient.* Because of a possible neck injury, do not place patient in the recovery position. Rather, hold the patient's head and neck in a straight position. If the patient vomits, turn his or her head, neck, and back to the side as single unit to let vomitus drain from the mouth. Continually reevaluate the patient for any change in status by assessing responsiveness, airway, breathing, and circulation every thirty seconds. Remember that the patient may fall back into cardiac arrest. Because the patient was just resuscitated from cardiac arrest, leave the AED in place. *Do not use the AED to reanalyze the patient's heart unless your assessment reveals that the patient has gone back into cardiac arrest.* Wait with the patient until advanced care arrives.

If the patient relapses into cardiac arrest, utilize the AED as previously described.

Scenario 7

In this scenario, the patient enters a state of nonshockable cardiac arrest after four defibrillating shocks. After one minute of CPR, the patient converts back into shockable cardiac arrest. Following the delivery of a fifth shock, the patient regains a pulse and adequate breathing. Prior to the successful defibrillation, the following emergency care must be given:

1. *Obtain the AED.* Quickly obtain the AED and move toward the patient's location. The dispatcher has already requested advanced care assistance.
2. *Size up the scene.* Ensure a safe scene and take BSI measures (gloves and protective face and eyewear). Quickly scan the patient for signs of a possible neck injury. In this scenario, you find no such signs.
3. *Assess the patient and prepare the AED.* Instruct your partner to determine unresponsiveness by shaking the patient and shouting, "Are you okay?" The patient is unresponsive. Since the patient is in a car, further assessment and care cannot be properly given. Therefore, remove the patient from the car to the ground of the parking lot. Prepare the AED for possible use. Have your partner complete the assessment by performing the following steps, in the order listed:
   - Check the patient's airway. Open the airway by performing the head tilt–chin lift maneuver.
   - Check the patient's breathing. Look, listen, and feel for breathing. The patient is breathless. Deliver two rescue breaths.
   - Check the patient's circulation. Check for a carotid pulse. No pulse is felt.

The patient is in cardiac arrest; therefore, fast application of the AED is critical. Since you have a partner to assist you, delegate all tasks not directly associated with the AED and its operation. Perform these steps, in this order:

4. *Initiate CPR.* Instruct your partner to initiate CPR. *As AED operator, do not stop preparation of the AED to assist with CPR!* This will delay the application of the AED.
5. *Apply the AED.* Turn on the AED and apply the electrodes to the patient's chest.
6. *Analyze the patient's heart.* Stop CPR and clear your partner from the patient. Press the ANALYZE button to analyze the patient's heart. A "SHOCK" message is received.
7. *Deliver a shock.* Ensure that your partner is clear of the patient, and press the SHOCK button to deliver the first shock.
8. *Reanalyze the patient's heart.* Do not check for a pulse, but immediately reanalyze the patient's heart. A "SHOCK" message is received.
9. *Deliver another shock.* Ensure that your partner is clear of the patient, and press the SHOCK button to deliver the second shock.
10. *Reanalyze the patient's heart.* Do not check for a pulse, but immediately reanalyze the patient's heart. A "SHOCK" message is received.

11. *Deliver a third shock.* Ensure that your partner is clear of the patient, and press the SHOCK button to deliver the third and final shock of the first set.

A full set of three stacked shocks has been delivered. Before performing additional analysis, one minute of CPR is needed to perfuse the body's cells with oxygen-rich blood. Continue with the following care:

12. *Check the patient's pulse.* Check for a carotid pulse. No pulse is felt. State "No pulse present. The patient is still in cardiac arrest!"
13. *Perform CPR.* Instruct your partner to perform CPR for one minute.
14. *Reanalyze the heart.* Stop CPR after one minute and clear your partner from the patient. Do not check for a pulse, but immediately reanalyze the patient's heart. A "SHOCK" message is received.
15. *Deliver a fourth shock.* Ensure that all providers are clear of the patient, and press the SHOCK button to deliver a fourth shock.
16. *Reanalyze the heart.* Do not check for a pulse, but immediately reanalyze the patient's heart. A "NO SHOCK" message is received.
17. *Check the patient's pulse.* Check for a carotid pulse. No pulse is felt. State, *"No pulse is present. The patient is in nonshockable cardiac arrest!"*
18. *Administer CPR.* Instruct your partner to perform CPR for one minute.
19. *Reanalyze the patient's heart.* Stop CPR after one minute and clear your partner from the patient. Do not check for a pulse, but immediately reanalyze the patient's heart. A "SHOCK" message is received. State, "The patient has converted to shockable cardiac arrest!"
20. *Deliver a fifth shock.* Ensure that your partner is clear of the patient, and press the SHOCK button to deliver a fifth shock.
21. *Reanalyze the heart.* Do not check for a pulse, but immediately reanalyze the patient's heart. A "NO SHOCK" message is received.
22. *Check the patient's pulse.* Check for a carotid pulse. A pulse is felt! State, "The patient has regained a pulse and is no longer in cardiac arrest!"

As the patient has regained a pulse, continue emergency care as follows:

23. *Check the patient's breathing.* Assess for breathing. In addition to having a pulse, the patient is breathing adequately. (If the patient were not breathing, you would administer rescue breaths at a rate of twelve per minute.)
24. *Place the patient in the recovery position.* Place the patient in the recovery position, as describe previously.
25. *Reassess the patient.* Continually reevaluate the patient for any change in status by assessing responsiveness, airway, breathing, and circulation every thirty seconds. Remember that the patient may fall back into cardiac arrest.

Because the patient was just resuscitated from cardiac arrest, leave the AED in place. *Do not use the AED to reanalyze the patient's heart unless your assessment reveals that the patient has gone back into cardiac arrest!* If it is available, administer oxygen via a face mask. Wait with the patient until advanced care arrives.

If the patient relapses into cardiac arrest, utilize the AED as previously described.

9

Death and Dying

Unsuccessful resuscitation—A rescue attempt in which a cardiac arrest patient dies despite all efforts to save his or her life.

Emotional difficulties—Difficulties in coping with the death of a cardiac arrest patient(s).

Methods of coping—Methods used by the health care provider to resolve feelings of emotional difficulty.

Despite your best efforts, some cardiac arrest patients will die. The death of a patient can spark frustration or even self-defeating attitudes or behaviors. You may question your delivery of care or experience emotional difficulties that disrupt your daily life. This chapter discusses the emotional impact of the death of a patient. Because of the nature of this material, there are no learning objectives for this chapter.

LIFE, DEATH, AND CARDIAC ARREST RESUSCITATION

There is no greater feeling than that of saving a life! Successfully resuscitating a person from cardiac arrest produces an exhilarating sense of wonder and achievement. A successful resuscitation is something of which you should be very proud. In emergency cardiac care, saving a life is the ultimate payoff.

Unfortunately, some victims of cardiac arrest are not successfully resuscitated. Even when the Chain of Survival is strong, some hearts are too sick, too old, or too weak to be restarted. Some patients have simply reached the natural end of life. *Consequently, the rescuer must understand that despite the most heroic of resuscitation efforts, some cardiac arrest patients will die.*

Nevertheless, an unsuccessful resuscitation can take an emotional toll on the rescuers providing emergency cardiac care. Some may experience a negative impact on their mental attitude and physical well-being. Other rescuers may begin to question the effectiveness of emergency cardiac care and develop the cynical belief that "it doesn't make a difference." Occasionally, the care provided by these individuals may become lackadaisical or even downright inappropriate.

Rescuers may unnecessarily burden themselves with feelings of guilt or responsibility—even when nothing more could have been done. These overwhelming feelings may lead to mistakes, confusion, and loss of control in future resuscitation efforts. If ignored, these feelings may spill over into a rescuer's personal life, affecting not only the rescuer but also his or her family and friends.

A cardiac arrest patient's best chance for survival depends on the quick delivery of quality cardiac care. Although some patients will die, *others will live if given the opportunity!* It is for these patients that rescuers must come to terms with their feelings and retain faith in the efficacy of emergency cardiac care. *A positive attitude on the part of a rescuer may very well mean the difference between life and death for the patient.*

COPING WITH DEATH

Coping with death requires the rescuer to recognize emotional difficulty and resolve it on an individual basis. Following are some methods of coping that may help rescuers and teams emotionally troubled by a patient's death.

- *Remain self-aware.* Recognizing signs of emotional difficulty is the most important part of coping with patient death. Irritability, difficulty sleeping, guilt, depression, and a general loss of interest may be signals indicating emotional difficulty.
- *Talk with team members.* Talking with other emergency cardiac care providers is another way to resolve troubling feelings. You may find that others have similar feelings and can provide helpful advice for coping. Comfort is often found in numbers.
- *Provide encouragement.* Encourage coworkers who appear in need of support. Become a listener, and give positive feedback without dwelling on the negative.
- *Critique past resuscitation efforts.* Hold critiques to discuss past resuscitation efforts. Critiques serve two purposes. First, critiques provide the opportunity to discuss personal feelings. Again, you may find that others

have similar feelings and can provide encouragement or advice related to coping. Second, critiques enable the team to reinforce positive aspects of care while identifying areas in need of improvement.

If feelings of emotional difficulty persist and begin to affect your daily life or cause physical problems like chest pain or headaches, it may be wise to consult a mental health professional.

SUMMARY

Not every cardiac arrest patient can be successfully resuscitated. Despite the most heroic of efforts, some cardiac arrest patients will die. For some rescuers, this lack of success can cause emotional difficulty.

Disregarding emotional difficulty can cause a self-defeating attitude and bring about both mental and physical problems for the rescuer. These problems may even spill into a rescuer's personal life. Mechanisms for coping with emotional stress are often beneficial for the emergency caregiver.

It is extremely important that the rescuer avoid becoming cynical or dissuaded from continuing the delivery of emergency cardiac care. *With the AED, the chance of saving lives is greater than ever before!* Remember that patient survival is strongly linked to quality emergency cardiac care—the kind of care an emotionally healthy caregiver delivers.

FOOD FOR THOUGHT

To test your understanding, read and discuss the following questions.

1. *After several unsuccessful resuscitation efforts, you have noticed yourself becoming increasingly irritable and sleepless at night. With no physical cause obvious, you suspect emotional difficulty related to the death of your patients. What are additional signs of emotional distress, and what measures can you take to resolve these feelings?*

   Aside from irritability and sleeplessness, signs of emotional difficulty include feelings of guilt, depression, and a general loss of interest in activities that once were very pleasurable. Recognizing that emotional difficulty exists is the first and most important step toward resolving it. Talking or gaining the support of other rescuers can help you resolve this situation. You may find that others have similar feelings. If such feelings spill over into your personal life or cause physical problems, consider consulting a mental health professional.

2. *You have noticed that a fellow emergency caregiver has become extremely depressed and guilt-ridden after the loss of a cardiac arrest patient. What are some ways you can help your team member?*

There are several ways you can help a rescuer who appears to be suffering from emotional difficulty related to patient death. Constantly look for the signs of such emotional difficulty, not only in others but also in yourself. Talking with a troubled rescuer may provide the release that he or she needs to begin the process of resolving these feelings. Provide encouragement that focuses on the positive aspects of the job rather than the negative ones.

3. *Critiquing previous resuscitation efforts is an important activity in relation to emotional coping. How can such critiques be beneficial?*

Critiquing past resuscitation efforts, both successful ones and unsuccessful ones, allows all involved to discuss feelings of emotional difficulty or other distressful feelings. Many times, comfort is gained in knowing that others have similar feelings. In this sense, critiques may provide encouragement to those in need and help them resolve negative feelings.

10

Special Topics

LEARNING OBJECTIVES

At the end of this chapter, you will be able to

- Describe the need for and essential nature of medical direction and written protocols
- Identify the need for and importance of skill maintenance
- Describe the importance of AED maintenance programs
- Describe the function of quality assurance

KEY TERMS

Initial training—A certified course in which the operation of the AED and other aspects of emergency cardiac care are learned and practiced.

Medical director—A physician responsible for all aspects of care given with an AED.

Skill maintenance—Continual practice of skills necessary for emergency cardiac care with an AED.

Documentation—Recording the events of a cardiac arrest resuscitation. Documentation occurs in written, audio, or computerized form.

Quality assurance—An organized process for identifying and evaluating areas of strong and weak performance in relation to emergency cardiac care.

When it is used quickly and appropriately, the AED can be a life-saving device. As the previous chapters have made clear, the operator of an AED must understand how to use the device and how to handle a variety of patient care situations. In addition to these aspects of providing emergency cardiac care, there are several considerations beyond the actual use of the device that contribute to providing effective emergency cardiac care with an AED. These "special topics" are discussed in this chapter.

INITIAL OPERATOR TRAINING

Before you can use an AED, you must complete a certified **initial training** program recognized by the state in which you wish to deliver care. The American Heart Association (AHA), National Safety Council, and American Red Cross have all developed quality AED training courses.

To take a course that deals exclusively with the AED, you should have preexisting certification in CPR and other basic life support techniques. AED training programs should cover all of the material discussed in this book.

MEDICAL DIRECTION AND PROTOCOLS

Completing an AED training course does not by itself permit you to freely use an AED. Since the AED is a medical device used to deliver medical care, you must practice under a physician, who acts as your **medical director**. State regulations dictate which physicians can and cannot function as a medical director.

A medical director is responsible for ensuring that emergency care delivered with an AED under his or her watch is provided in a safe and effective manner. Because it is physically impossible for a medical director to be present at every cardiac arrest, he or she issues **protocols**.

Protocols are written policies and procedures that outline how you are to deliver emergency cardiac care with an AED. All rescuers using an AED must abide by written protocols. If you do not follow the written protocols, disciplinary action and legal liability will follow—even if the patient is not harmed! *Consequently, protocols must be followed without exception!*

Because a medical director is accountable for the entire scope of care under his or her watch, the director's responsibilities go beyond the use of an AED to encompass such things as administrative issues related to AEDs and so on. Such responsibilities include the following:

- Designating the type of AED to be used
- Authorizing who can and cannot use the AED

- Ensuring competency among those authorized to use the AED
- Setting guidelines on training and skill review and on emergency cardiac care
- Determining the type of data storage and documentation needed

In addition, the medical director (or assigned designee) should review every cardiac arrest incident to ensure that appropriate care was delivered.

SKILL MAINTENANCE

To stay sharp and maintain the skills needed to deliver quality care with an AED, it is recommended that you take an AED refresher class every three to six months (American Heart Association, 1998). At a minimum, a refresher class should include the following:

- Critique of previous cardiac arrest resuscitations
- Review of AED operation and maintenance guidelines
- Review of AED protocols
- Hands-on practice with the AED

Many AED manufacturers offer a training simulator that can be connected to a CPR mannequin. These simulators provide true-to-life cardiac arrest simulations that must be treated as if real. Patient assessment, CPR, defibrillation, and safety measures should also be reviewed.

AED MAINTENANCE

Proper maintenance is critical for proper operation! Inappropriate or neglected maintenance can lead to AED malfunction and the possibility of injury to both patient and rescuer. To avoid medical and legal problems, regular maintenance is necessary.

AED manufacturers issue strict guidelines for preventive maintenance. Many of the newer AEDs conduct an internal check and signal you when a problem is discovered.

The primary cause of AED malfunction is battery failure! Batteries should be maintained per manufacturer's instructions and recharged or replaced when needed. In addition, fully charged spare batteries should be available at all times for emergency use.

Using a checklist can help you spot other potential problems. Completing a checklist requires that you examine the AED and ensure that all supplies are

AUTOMATED DEFIBRILLATORS: OPERATOR'S SHIFT CHECKLIST

Date: _____   Shift: _____   Location: _____

Mfr/Model No.: _____   Serial No. or Facility ID No.: _____

At the beginning of each shift, inspect the unit. Indicate whether all requirements have been met. Note any corrective actions taken. Sign the form.

	Okay as found	Corrective Action/Remarks
1. Defibrillator Unit		
Clean no spills, clear of objects on top, casing intact		
2. Cables/Connectors		
a. Inspect for cracks, broken wire, or damage b. Connectors engage securely		
3. Supplies		
a. Two sets of pads in sealed packages, within expiration date b. Hand towel c. Scissors d. Razor * e. Alcohol wipes * f. Monitoring electrodes *g. Spare charged battery *h. Adequate ECG paper *i. Manual override module, key or card *j. Cassette tape, memory module, and/or event card plus spares		
4. Power Supply		
a. Battery-powered units (1) Verify fully charged battery in place (2) Spare charged battery available (3) Follow appropriate battery rotation schedule per manufacturer's recommendations b. AC/Battery backup units (1) Plugged into live outlet to maintain battery charge (2) Test on battery power and reconnect to line power		
5. Indicators/*ECG Display		
* a. Remove cassette tape, memory module, and/or event card b. Power on display c. Self-test ok * d. Monitor display functional *e. "Service" message display off *f. Battery charging; low battery light off g. Correct time displayed — set with dispatch center		
6. ECG Recorder		
a. Adequate ECG paper b. Recorder prints		
7. Charge/Display Cycle		
* a. Disconnect AC plug — battery backup units b. Attach to simulator c. Detects, charges and delivers shock for "VF" d. Responds correctly to non-shockable rhythms *e. Manual override functional f. Detach from simulator *g. Replace cassette tape, module, and/or memory card		
8. *Pacemaker		
a. Pacer output cable intact b. Pacer pads present (set of two) c. Inspect per manufacturer's operational guidelines		
☐ **Major problem(s) identified** (OUT OF SERVICE)		

*Applicable only if the unit has this supply or capability

Signature: _____

Figure 10–1   Sample AED Maintenance Checklist (*Source:* Hafen, Karren, & Mistovich, 1996, p. 322)

present and that the machine is functional. See Figure 10–1 for a sample checklist. Checklists help identify problems before the device is needed.

When a problem is identified, follow the manufacturer's recommendations for repair. Never attempt to fix a problem you are not authorized to address. *Repairs must be made only by persons officially certified in AED repair!*

AED MALFUNCTION AND THE MEDWATCH PROGRAM

The Safe Medical Devices Act of 1990 requires that all accidents involving the use of an AED be reported. Through the Medwatch program, any injury or death in which an AED was a contributing factor must be officially registered. The Medwatch program was established by the FDA to ensure the safety of all regulated medical devices (American Heart Association, 1997).

DOCUMENTATION

Documentation is an important but often overlooked aspect of emergency cardiac care. Documentation provides a record of all events that occur during the delivery of emergency care.

As discussed previously, most AEDs have an audio recorder with which the AED operator can record a narration of the entire cardiac arrest resuscitation effort. Additionally, most AEDs have a computerized memory module that automatically records the state of the cardiac arrest patient's heart, defibrillations, and response to the defibrillations. Additionally, the AED checklist is a form of documentation.

The AED operator must also provide written documentation of each rescue effort. This should be completed on a specialized form. When documenting a cardiac arrest resuscitation, you should document the entire incident, from notification or discovery to the transfer of care to another medical authority. All patient care and interventions, and the time you performed them, must be noted. Figure 10–2 illustrates an AED documentation form.

Documentation is an important tool in evaluating the effectiveness of emergency cardiac care. Additionally, documentation can provide research data. All documentation should be saved for possible audit or legal needs.

QUALITY ASSURANCE

Quality assurance is the administrative function that evaluates performance. Quality assurance examines each cardiac arrest, scrutinizing weak areas while

(Circle correct response Y or N)

Service Name: _____   Address: _____

Medical Director: _____

Patient Name: _____   Address: _____

_____ TIMES: _____   _____ FATE FACTORS: _____

Time of call: _____   1st Defib: _____

Dispatch: _____   2nd Defib: _____

Scene arrival: _____   3rd Defib: _____

Hosp arrival: _____   CPR started: _____

_____ PERFORMANCE VARIABLES: _____

Witnessed arrest:	(Y)	(N)
Time of arrest:	(_____	)
CPR prior to arrival:	(Y)	(N)
Sex of patient:	(M)	(F)
Hx of previous arrest:	(Y)	(N)
Hx of heart trouble:	(Y)	(N)
Heart meds:	(Y)	(N)
Rhythm on arrival:	(Y)	(N)

First shock energy setting: _____   Resultant rhythm: _____
                                            Pulse present   (Y)   (N)

Second shock energy setting: _____   Resultant rhythm: _____
                                            Pulse present   (Y)   (N)

Third shock energy setting: _____   Resultant rhythm: _____
                                            Pulse present   (Y)   (N)

Airway established by EMTs   ALS personnel
  Manual (Y)   Oral (Y)   Nasal (Y)   ET (Y)   Other (Y) _____

Spontaneous breathing began (Y) (N)   Time: _____   Oxygen: (Y)   LPM: ( )

_____ PATIENT OUTCOME: _____

Hospital arrival: Rhythm: _____

Pulse (Y) (N)   Spontaneous breathing (Y) (N)

Admitted to hospital (Y) (N)   Discharged alive (Y) (N)

How many days to discharge (alive or expired): _____

Form completed by: (Print) _____

          (Signature) _____

Date: _____

ECG strips must be attached   Mail to:
Transcription must be attached

Figure 10–2   Sample Written Documentation Form   (*Source:* Weigle, Atkins, & Taylor, 1988, p. 60)

reinforcing strong performance. It assesses not only the use of the AED but also the entire Chain of Survival. If problems with performance are identified, corrective action must be taken. All forms of documentation are invaluable in the quality assurance process. Since the medical director reviews all rescue efforts, he or she plays a crucial role in quality assurance.

SUMMARY

Aside from the correct physical use of the AED, quality emergency care depends on other, less apparent considerations such as those discussed in this chapter. An improperly maintained AED or an emergency care system that does not have a quality assurance process compromises the overall effectiveness of care. Likewise, poor documentation or deficient **skill maintenance** represents a direct threat to quality patient care and patient survival.

Successful resuscitation of a cardiac arrest patient depends on fast delivery of quality care. Quality care cannot be delivered when these special topics are neglected or considered unimportant. To give the cardiac arrest patient the highest chance for survival, these special topics must be considered as important as the procedures for operating the AED.

FOOD FOR THOUGHT

To test your understanding, read and discuss the following questions.

1. *You are a certified AED care provider with a volunteer fire department in a sparsely populated rural county. You typically handle one or two cardiac arrests per year. Why is attending an AED refresher course every three to six months important?*

Proper use of the AED depends on the rescuer's staying proficient in skills like patient assessment, CPR, operation of the AED, and medical care given when the AED is successful or unsuccessful in restoring a heartbeat. Without continual practice and reinforcement, these skills may quickly fade from memory—especially when they are not used on a routine basis. Therefore, it is important to attend AED refresher classes at regular intervals.

In an AED refresher class, the skills necessary for resuscitating a patient and operating an AED are reviewed. Review of AED operation and hands-on practice are invaluable for skill maintenance. Critiques of previous rescue efforts add to the overall learning process. AED refresher courses are necessary to maintain the skills and knowledge necessary to deliver quality care. It is this quality care that gives the patient the best chance for survival.

2. *As an AED provider in a local medical clinic, you are approached by a woman wishing to start an AED program in her office building. She asks what type of initial training is needed and whether or not a medical director is necessary. How would you answer her?*

When starting an AED program, you must secure the backing of a physician to act as a medical director. Remember that the AED is a medical device, and as such it cannot be used without the permission of a doctor. Many states have regulations that dictate which physicians can and cannot serve as an AED medical director.

In addition, all rescuers must take a certified AED course. The American Heart Association, the National Safety Council, and the American Red Cross are highly regarded organizations that offer AED courses. It is also important for rescuers to have existing certification in CPR if CPR certification is not included in the AED course.

3. *Your medical director has appointed you his quality assurance assistant. What is quality assurance, and what responsibilities will you have as a quality assurance officer?*

Quality assurance is an administrative function that makes sure the quality of care given with an AED meets established standards. Quality assurance is the organized process of examining all aspects of emergency cardiac care, with the goal of identifying strong and weak areas. Strong performance can be reinforced and weak areas improved on.

In addition to actual operation of the AED, quality assurance encompasses other areas such as documentation, patient assessment, response times, personnel availability, and the Chain of Survival as a whole. Consequently, quality assurance is an important part of emergency cardiac care.

4. *Documentation is an important part of providing emergency cardiac care. What different forms of documentation are used with an AED, and why is thorough documentation important?*

Documenting all of the events of a cardiac arrest resuscitation effort is an invaluable step in the quality assurance process. In addition, documentation may be required at a later time for medical or legal needs.

Documentation comes in different forms. Using a special documentation sheet, rescuers must provide a complete written account of the entire incident, from notification to transfer of care, for every patient—even if the effort was unsuccessful or the AED was not used.

So Whatever Became of John Maynerd?

A police officer quickly arrived with an AED. After performing a patient assessment and confirming cardiac arrest, the officer quickly applied the AED electrodes to John's chest. The AED returned a "SHOCK" message, and John was promptly defibrillated. After the first defibrillation, a "NO SHOCK" message was received. The police officer checked for a carotid pulse and located one, albeit weak. At the same time, the female bank patron noticed John's hand moving. Although John was not fully conscious, he would open his eyes when told to do so. He was placed in the recovery position.

Paramedics arrived with equipment to render advanced care. A tube was quickly placed into John's windpipe, through which ventilations and oxygen were supplied. An IV line was initiated, through which fluids and emergency medications were administered. The AED did not allow viewing of John's ECG, so the paramedics attached their cardiac monitor defibrillator to him.

The paramedics brought in the cot from the ambulance and secured John to it. Once he was in place, they wheeled him to the ambulance and took him quickly to a hospital five miles from the bank. Remarkably, John did indeed survive and was discharged two weeks later. He never did make the surprise party, but his second chance at life was more than his wife could ever have asked for.

This is a true story. I was one of the paramedics who helped care for John. He survived because of a strong Chain of Survival and community support. If it had not been for the bank teller's acquiring early access, the woman's performing CPR, and the police officer's administering early defibrillation, John would never have made it out of that bank alive. With a strong Chain of Survival and a commitment to AEDs on the part of local communities, there will be many stories like this to tell.

Also, many AEDs contain an audio recorder to record a verbal account by the AED operator. Additionally, most AEDs have a computerized module that records data such as changes in the heart rhythm, number of defibrillations, and patient response to defibrillations for download at a later time. Even the AED checklist and maintenance log are forms of medical documentation.

REFERENCES

American Heart Association. (1997). *Basic life support for healthcare providers.* Dallas: Author.

American Heart Association. (1998). *Heartsaver AED for the lay rescuer and first responder.* Dallas: Author.

Karren, K. J., Hafen, B. Q., & Limmer, D. (1998). *First responder: A skills approach* (5th ed.) Upper Saddle River, NJ: Prentice Hall/Brady.

Weigel, A., Atkins, J. M., & Taylor, J. (1988). Automated defibrillation. Englewood, CO: Morton.

Appendix A:
Adult Rescue Breathing

Perform adult rescue breathing once you determine that the patient is breathless but has a pulse.

MOUTH-TO-MOUTH RESCUE BREATHING

1. Open the patient's airway.
   - Use the head tilt–chin lift if there is no evidence of a possible traumatic neck injury.
   - Use the jaw-thrust maneuver if there is evidence of traumatic neck injury.
2. Gently pinch the patient's nose shut.
3. Seal your lips around the patient's mouth to create an airtight seal.
4. Deliver twelve rescue breaths per minute (1 breath every 5 seconds).

RESCUE BREATHING WITH A POCKET MASK

1. Position the pocket mask over the patient's mouth and nose:
   - Create a seal by placing your thumb and index finger on each side of the mask.
   - Place your remaining fingers along the bottom of the patient's jaw.
   - Tilt the patient's head backward to maintain the open airway (only if the patient has not sustained a traumatic neck injury). Use the jaw thrust maneuver if you suspect a traumatic neck injury.

2. Place your mouth over the one-way valve of the pocket mask.
3. Deliver twelve rescue breaths per minute (1 breath every 5 seconds) (American Heart Association, 1997).

REFERENCE

American Heart Association. (1997). *Basic life support heartsaver guide—A student handbook for cardiopulmonary resuscitation and first aid for choking.* Dallas: Author.

Appendix B:
Adult Cardiopulmonary Resuscitation

ADULT ONE-RESCUER CPR

1. Establish unresponsiveness and access the EMS system.
2. Open the patient's airway.
   - Use the head tilt–chin lift maneuver if there is no evidence of a possible traumatic neck injury.
   - Use the jaw-thrust maneuver if you suspect a traumatic neck injury.
3. Check the patient's breathing. Look, listen, and feel for breathing.
   - If there is no breathing, deliver two slow rescue breaths.
   - If the first rescue breath does not pass through to the patient's lungs, reposition the patient's head and reattempt the rescue breath.
   - If the second rescue breath does not pass through, assume there is a foreign body airway obstruction (see Appendix C).
   - If the patient is breathing and displays no evidence of a possible traumatic neck injury, place the patient in the recovery position.
   - If the patient is breathing and you suspect a possible traumatic neck injury, hold the head, neck, and back in a straight position while maintaining the jaw thrust maneuver to keep the airway open. If the patient vomits, turn his or her head, neck, and back to the side so the vomitus drains from the mouth.
4. Check the patient's circulation. Check for a carotid pulse.
   - If there is no pulse, start CPR (chest compressions and rescue breaths). Perform a cycle of fifteen chest compressions followed by two rescue breaths at a rate of eighty to one hundred per minute.
   - If a pulse is present, start rescue breathing (see Appendix A).

5. After one minute of CPR, again check for a carotid pulse.
   - If there is still no pulse, continue cycles of fifteen chest compressions followed by two rescue breaths.
   - If a pulse is present, start rescue breathing (see Appendix A).
6. If the patient is breathing and displays no evidence of a possible traumatic neck injury, place the patient into the recovery position.

If the patient is breathing and you suspect a possible traumatic neck injury, hold the head, neck, and back in a straight position while maintaining the jaw thrust maneuver to keep the airway open. If the patient vomits, turn his or her head, neck, and back to the side so that the vomitus drains from the mouth (American Heart Association, 1997).

Adult Two-Rescuer CPR

In adult two-rescuer CPR, the first rescuer performs the ABCs of patient assessment. If the patient is in cardiac arrest, the first rescuer provides rescue breathing while the second rescuer delivers chest compressions.

1. Establish unresponsiveness and access the EMS system. The first rescuer performs the following:
2. Open the patient's airway.
   - Use the head tilt–chin lift maneuver if there is no evidence of possible traumatic neck injury.
   - Use the jaw-thrust maneuver if you suspect a traumatic neck injury.
3. Check the patient's breathing. Look, listen, and feel for breathing.
   - If the patient is not breathing, deliver two slow rescue breaths.
   - If the first breath does not pass through to the lungs, reposition the patient's head and reattempt the rescue breath.
   - If the second rescue breath does not pass through, assume there is a foreign body airway obstruction (see Appendix C).
   - If the patient is breathing and displays no evidence of a possible traumatic neck injury, place the patient in the recovery position.
   - If the patient is breathing and you suspect a possible traumatic neck injury, hold the head, neck, and back in a straight position while maintaining the jaw thrust maneuver to keep the airway open. If the patient vomits, turn his or her head, neck, and back to the side so that the vomitus drains from the mouth.
4. Check the patient's circulation. Check for a carotid pulse.
   - If there is no pulse, start CPR.
   - If a pulse is present, start rescue breathing if needed (see Appendix A).

The first and second rescuers then perform the following:

5. Deliver five chest compressions (second rescuer), followed by one rescue breath (first rescuer).
6. Repeat cycles of five chest compressions followed by one rescue breath for one minute.
7. After one minute of CPR, check for a carotid pulse.
   • If there is still no pulse, continue cycles of five chest compressions followed by one rescue breath.
   • If a pulse is present, start rescue breathing if needed (see Appendix A).
8. If the patient is breathing and displays no evidence of a possible traumatic neck injury, place the patient in the recovery position.

If the patient is breathing and you suspect a possible traumatic neck injury, hold the head, neck, and back in a straight position while maintaining the jaw thrust maneuver to keep the airway open. If the patient vomits, turn the head, neck, and back to the side so that the vomitus drains from the mouth (American Heart Association, 1997).

REFERENCE

American Heart Association. (1997). *Basic life support heartsaver guide—A student handbook for cardiopulmonary resuscitation and first aid for choking.* Dallas: Author.

Appendix C:
Unresponsive with a Foreign
Body Airway Obstruction

When attempts to deliver two rescue breaths to an unresponsive, nonbreathing patient are unsuccessful, you should suspect a foreign body airway obstruction.

1. Open the patient's mouth and perform a blind finger sweep.
2. If the blind finger sweep does not clear the obstruction, perform abdominal thrusts with the patient in a lying position.
   - Place the heel of your hand on the patient's abdomen, just above the navel but below the end of the sternum.
   - Place your other hand on top of the first.
   - Deliberately thrust your hands into the patient's abdomen in an inward and upward motion, up to five times.
3. Open the patient's mouth with the tongue jaw lift and perform a blind finger sweep.
4. Attempt two rescue breaths.
5. Administer up to five abdominal thrusts.
6. Repeat Steps 3 through 5 until the foreign body airway obstruction is expelled and attempts at rescue breaths are successful (American Heart Association, 1997).

REFERENCE

American Heart Association. (1997). *Basic life support heartsaver guide—A student handbook for cardiopulmonary resuscitation and first aid for choking.* Dallas: Author.

Glossary

ABC—For the ABCs of assessment; after determining unresponsiveness, check the patient's airway, breathing, and circulation.

Acute myocardial infarction—The most common form of cardiac compromise; occurs when heart cells are deprived of oxygen and begin to die.

Advanced care—Procedures like controlling the patient's airway, administering IV fluids or drugs, and defibrillation if it has not yet been performed.

Analysis—The process by which an AED evaluates the condition of a person's heart and decides whether the heart is shockable or nonshockable.

Arteries—Large blood vessels that bring oxygenated blood to the cells of the body.

Asystole—See *Flat-line condition.*

Automated external defibrillator (AED)—A device capable of delivering defibrillation automatically, requiring little or no training to operate.

Automated implantable cardiac defibrillator (AICD)—A small defibrillator that is internally attached to the wall of the heart.

Basic life support—Basic measures to support life. Basic life support includes opening the airway, performing rescue breathing, and performing CPR.

Biphasic defibrillation—Defibrillation in which the electrical current is reversed halfway through the shock.

Body substance isolation—Measures taken to limit the transmission of infectious diseases.

Capillaries—The tiny blood vessels that lie next to cells.

Cardiac arrest—The condition in which the heart stops pumping blood.

Cardiac arrest resuscitation—The process of delivering emergency care to a cardiac arrest patient.

Cardiac compromise—A condition in which there is a problem with the heart and its ability to pump blood.

Cardiac pacemaker—A mechanical device that electrically stimulates the heart to beat and pump blood.

Cardiopulmonary resuscitation (CPR)—Delivery of rescue breathing and chest compressions for a person in cardiac arrest.

Carotid artery—The most reliable artery for determining the presence or absence of a pulse.

Cells—Tiny living building blocks that make up all human beings. All cells require oxygen for survival.

Chain of Survival—A sequence, developed by the American Heart Association, consisting of the four critical actions (links in the chain) that must be taken to give a cardiac arrest patient the best chance for survival.

Communication system—The part of the AED that permits it to communicate with the rescuer.

Data recording system—An audio or electronic component of an AED that permits documentation of a cardiac arrest incident while the AED is being used.

Defibrillation—The controlled delivery of electrical shocks to a heart in cardiac arrest. Frequently, early defibrillation serves to restart the heart and enable it to pump blood.

Defibrillator—A device that delivers a defibrillating shock.

Documentation—Recording the events of a cardiac arrest resuscitation. Documentation occurs in written, audio, or computerized form.

Electrodes—Adhesive pads that attach to a patient's chest and are connected by cables to an AED.

Electrocardiogram (ECG)—The heart's electrical tracing.

Emotional difficulties—Difficulties in coping with the death of a cardiac arrest patient.

Flat-line condition—The nonshockable state of cardiac arrest; signifies a dead heart.

Fully automated external defibrillator (FAED)—An AED that automatically analyzes the heart and delivers a defibrillating shock without any operator input.

Head tilt–chin lift maneuver—Procedure to clear the airway of patients not suspected of having suffered a traumatic spinal injury.

Heart—A fist-sized muscular organ that pumps blood throughout the body.

Heart attack—See *acute myocardial infarction.*

Hypothermia—A state in which the internal body temperature is below normal.

Infectious disease—A transmittable disease that can cause infection of the rescuer.

Initial training—A certified course in which the operation of the AED and other aspects of emergency cardiac care are learned and practiced.

Jaw-thrust maneuver—Procedure for opening the airway of a patient suspected of having suffered traumatic neck injury.

Medical director—A physician responsible for all aspects of care given with an AED.

Medication patch—A small patch containing medication that is absorbed through the skin.

Methods of coping—Methods used by the health care provider to resolve feelings of emotional difficulty associated with the death of a patient.

NO SHOCK message—The message displayed by an AED that has determined that a heart is in a nonshockable state and will not benefit from a defibrillating shock.

Nonshockable cardiac arrest—A state of cardiac arrest that will not benefit from a defibrillator shock.

Oxygen—Odorless, tasteless, colorless gas necessary for life.

Patient assessment—A systematic evaluation of a patient's level of responsiveness, airway, breathing, and circulation. A patient assessment quickly reveals the presence or absence of cardiac arrest.

Protocols—Written policies and procedures that outline how you are to deliver emergency cardiac care with an AED.

Quality assurance—An organized process for identifying and evaluating strong and weak areas in relation to emergency cardiac care.

Scene size-up—A quick evaluation of the scene of a cardiac arrest.

Semiautomated external defibrillator (SAED)—An AED that requires the operator to manually activate the analysis and defibrillating shock when advised to do so by the AED.

Shock advisory defibrillator—A semiautomated external defibrillator.

SHOCK message—The message displayed by an AED that has determined that a heart is in a shockable state and will benefit from a defibrillating shock.

Shockable cardiac arrest—A state of cardiac arrest that will benefit from early defibrillation.

Skill maintenance—Continual practice of skills necessary for emergency cardiac care with an AED.

Smart AEDs—AEDS that calculate the exact amount of electricity needed to successfully defibrillate a heart in shockable cardiac arrest.

Stacked shocks—A set of up to three shocks delivered consecutively by an AED as long as the heart is in a shockable state.

Sternum—The breastbone.

Traumatic injury—Any injury caused by force or energy.

Unsuccessful resuscitation—A rescue attempt in which a patient dies despite all efforts to save his or her life.

Veins—Large blood vessels that bring oxygen-poor blood back to the heart and lungs.

Ventricular fibrillation—A state in which the heart quivers weakly like a glob of gelatin.

Index

ABCs. *See* Patient assessment
Acute myocardial infarction (AMI), 5
Advanced care, 13, 62
  unavailability of, 70
AED. *See* Automated external
  defibrillator
Age guidelines, 68–69
Airway, 40–42
Analysis, 51
Analyze button, 27
Arteries, 5
Asystole, 18
Audio recorder, 29–30
Automated external defibrillator (AED)
  batteries, 28–29, 99
  chain of survival and, 13–14, 24
  components of, 26–30
  control panel, 27
  data recording systems, 23, 29–30
  defibrillation with, 13
  description, 11, 24
  effectiveness, 31
  electrodes and placement, 23, 27–28
  fully automated external defibrillator,
    23, 25
  maintenance, 99–101
  malfunction, 28, 99
  principles of use, 53–54

  semiautomated external defibrillator,
    23, 25
  types of, 25
Automated Implantable Cardiac
  Defibrillator (AICD), 67, 69–70

Basic life support, 35
  See also Cardiopulmonary
    resuscitation
Batteries, 28–29, 99
Biphasic defibrillation, 25–26
Blood circulation, 5
Blood vessels, 5
Body substance isolation (BSI), 35, 37
Breathing. *See* Patient Assessment
Breathlessness, 7, 42
BSI. *See* Body substance isolation

Cables, 27
Capillaries, 5
Cardiac arrest
  description, 3, 5
  nonshockable, 17, 18
  resuscitation, 52, 54–64
  shockable, 17, 18
  signs of, 7
  traumatic, 71
  ventricular fibrillation, 17, 18–19